Praise

JUST RUN

'Merili shares her running experiences with unflinching honesty and vulnerability, proving that running isn't just about finish lines – it's about embracing the journey, overcoming obstacles, and discovering our limitless potential.'

- LISA JACKSON, AUTHOR OF *YOUR PACE OR MINE?*

'Merili has managed to do what might seem beyond reach to most people. She has proven that it is not only possible to start running from the lowliest of places – from barely walking 3,000 steps a day during the Covid pandemic in 2020 to completing an ultra marathon just a handful of years later – but she has also shared her story skilfully and passionately in the pages of her new book, *Just Run*. In reading this book, I can see echoes of my own journey, not only with running but also with disordered eating, overcoming obstacles, including self-doubt and the fear of looking foolish. As somebody who knows how hard it is to tackle those fears head on, I can only applaud Merili for being brave enough to push herself far beyond her old self-imposed limits and create a new reality for herself, and then sharing her story so articulately with the world.'

- RACHEL ANN CULLEN, AUTHOR OF *RUNNING FOR MY LIFE*

'Merili Freear reminds us that running at its essence is quite simple: it's about getting outside and putting one foot in front of the other. The rest is discovery. And as you'll discover in her aptly named book, if you "just run", no matter how slowly or tentatively at first, a new world will open up before you.'

- JOHN HANC, AUTHOR OF *THE ESSENTIAL RUNNER* AND *THE COOLEST RACE ON EARTH*

'If you're struggling to start running, this memoir is the running buddy you need to get out there! *Just Run* is the encouragement to find joy in running without comparison and illustrates more is possible from running three times a week than you may have imagined.'

- RONNIE STATON, ULTRA RUNNER, COACH AND HOBO PACE RACE DIRECTOR

'It's a very honest book, and it's made me realise that a lot of things I personally worry about as a runner are things that also bother other people too, as I found myself nodding along to a lot of what Merili says in here. Merili overcomes obstacles – self-doubt, injury, lack of motivation – and helps the reader understand that we all experience these at some time or another, and that they are not insurmountable. Beginners would find this useful – there are lots of tips in there, as well as useful pace charts and mile/kilometre conversions. However, I've been running for many, many years and also found lots in there for me too – including an entire chapter dedicated to canicross, which I don't often see written about in books. I loved that the chapters are short, so it's a very easy book to dip in and out of, even if you only have 5 minutes to spare at a time. I am also a busy mum, like Merili, so appreciated this format. All in all, this is an inspiring read about all aspects of running, both positive and negative.'

- MICHELLE MORTIMER, UKRUNCHAT

'I thoroughly enjoyed this book, particularly as two of my favourite worlds collided: running and reading. Whether you're just thinking about running, are a beginner, or an experienced runner, there's something here for everyone.'

- SUSAN WHEATCROFT, VIRTUAL RUNNER UK

JUST RUN

DISCOVERING MY LOVE FOR RUNNING AND
HOW THE IMPOSSIBLE BECOMES POSSIBLE

MERILI FREEAR

First Edition 2024 *Just Run*

Copyright © Merili Freear, 2024

All rights reserved. No part of the publication may be reproduced, stored in a retrieval system, transmitted or circulated in any form or by any means, electronic, mechanical, photocopying, recording or otherwise, without prior permission in writing from the author. For permissions contact the author: meriliruns@gmail.com

Although every precaution has been taken to verify the accuracy of the information contained herein, the author assumes no responsibility for any errors or omissions. No liability is assumed for losses or damages that may result from the use of information contained within. You are responsible for your own choices, actions and results.

The author is not associated with any product or vendor mentioned in this book.

Every effort has been made to trace the copyright holders and obtain permission to reproduce material. Please do get in touch with any enquiries or any information relating to the rights holder.

A CIP catalogue record for this book is available from the British Library.

ISBN: 978-1-7385559-0-1 (paperback)
ISBN: 978-1-7385559-1-8 (hardcover)
ISBN: 978-1-7385559-9-4 (e-book)

Editor: Siân Smith
Cover design: Katarina Naskovski
Book design: Furkan Süperdoğan

The information in this book is not intended to be a substitute for the medical advice of a licensed physician. The reader should consult with their doctor in any matters relating to their health. Before beginning any exercise programme, it is recommended that you seek medical advice from your personal physician.

For Jacob,

Never stop believing in yourself or chasing your dreams. Remember that you can accomplish everything you put your heart into.

Foreword

Why do we run? How do we run? How could we run better? These are only a few of the many questions Merili Freear answers in her debut memoir, *Just Run: Discovering my love for running and how the impossible becomes possible.*

As an ultra marathoner, I generally relate to most runners. And when I began to follow Merili Freear on social media, I felt I'd found a new friend. From her love of dogs to her physical issues most won't say out loud, as well as the mental health challenges she navigates, I knew we were kindred spirits. She gets me!

In my first book, the running and mental health memoir, *Depression Hates a Moving Target: How Running with My Dog Brought Me Back from the Brink,* I shared my running story: the how, the why, the what. We might not even know why we start to run, but once we've felt the benefits the reason becomes clear: we're trying to save ourselves.

For Merili, that saving needed to happen during the pandemic. Amidst the turmoil, she craved quiet solitude; a temporary escape from the disorder the Covid-19 lockdown heaped on so many of us. But Merili knew she needed something more than just tranquillity: deep inside, she knew she was yearning for something that reminded her of her inner resilience. And so, she laced up and found a way to silence her insecurities, finding moments of clarity amidst the chaos.

Balancing the challenges of explaining the Covid-19 restrictions to her toddler, Merili discovered her passion for running. It's clear how her dedication to running not only made her a better wife and mother but also served as a lifeline during uncertain times. We are both fortunate to have great men at our sides; that constant and continuous cheerleader who understands the power of running (even if they don't run themselves!).

Merili shares her experience as a true beginner, as so many of us start out. But how many beginner runners end up training as running coaches? Merili's qualification as a running coach means you can benefit from the dual aspect of her experience: from her mistakes as a beginner to the wealth of knowledge and expertise she later learns as a trained running coach, which she passionately shares with you all.

Merili's intimate understanding of the impact of running on both physical and mental wellbeing, combined with her inclusive approach and coaching knowledge, makes her uniquely qualified to write this book.

If you're looking for inspiration, not just about running, but about overcoming life's challenges, *Just Run* is for you.

Nita Sweeney
Upper Arlington, Ohio, USA
April, 2024

Contents

Author's Note   13

Prologue   15

PART I: ZERO TO MARATHON   21

Chapter 1: That First Run   23

Chapter 2: My First Running Experiences and First Races   31

Chapter 3: Just Run   39

Chapter 4: I'm a Runner!   45

Chapter 5: Marathon?   53

Chapter 6: Eating Sticks and Leaves   59

Chapter 7: Taper Turmoil   67

Chapter 8: Part of 1%   75

Chapter 9: Aftermath of the Marathon   83

PART II: A YEAR OF SETBACKS — 89

Chapter 10: When Your Body Doesn't Work with You — 91

Chapter 11: Running Is Cheaper Than Therapy — 101

Chapter 12: Rebound — 107

Chapter 13: Back in the Game — 113

Chapter 14: Always a Lone Runner? — 119

Chapter 15: Virtual London Marathon — 125

Chapter 16: The Way Forward — 135

Chapter 17: Forced Running Break — 141

Chapter 18: Run the Thames — 147

Chapter 19: Forty Miles for My 40th — 153

Chapter 20: Dukeries — 163

PART III: MY RUNNING STYLE — 171

Chapter 21: Running Three Times a Week — 175

Chapter 22: Sunday, Runday — 181

Chapter 23: Half Marathons That Changed Me — 187

Chapter 24: Runner's High — 193

Chapter 25: Tackling the Dreadmill — 197

Chapter 26: From Virtual Racing to Racing — 201

Chapter 27: Little Goals Make You Feel Good — 207

Chapter 28: Running Group — 211

Chapter 29: Rain Rain Go Away Come Back Another Day — 215

Chapter 30: Canicross   221
Chapter 31: Glorious Holiday Running   227
Chapter 32: Inspiring Movies and Books   235
Chapter 33: My Top Tips   241
Chapter 34: Why Run?   271

Epilogue   275
Glossary   279
Appendix 1: Recommended Reading   285
Appendix 2: Miles vs Km   288
Appendix 3: Km vs Miles   289
Appendix 4: Race Pace   290
References   291
Acknowledgements   293
About the Author   296

Author's Note

I ran a marathon! I completed a full 26.2 miles! These were the thoughts that crossed my mind when I first considered writing a book. As I began writing, however, my usual imposter syndrome took over, and I questioned whether my marathon achievement had been a mere fluke. I wondered who would want to read about my struggles with running a marathon. People run marathons all the time, right?

I questioned whether I truly possessed the essence of a writer. Then it struck me – writing and running aren't so different after all. I decided to approach my writing in the same way as my running: taking those initial steps out of my comfort zone and embracing the challenge of something new.

Since my teenage years, I've harboured a desire to write a book, but the right time never seemed to come, or I felt I had little to say. It all seemed overwhelming. So, I started small. I took on a writing challenge for an entire month to nurture my creativity. Every morning, I wrote three pages of whatever came to my mind. Then, one particular morning, instead of my usual morning pages, I began writing bits of my book – bit by bit every day. That's how this book was born: just by believing that I could.

Feel free to read this book from cover to cover, or you can jump to part III to delve into my running style and find tips for beginner runners. Parts I and II are best read in chronological order.

I am originally from Estonia, where the metric system is prevalent. Consequently, I prefer measuring my runs in kilometres (abbreviated to 'k', hence 5k and 10k), though since living in the UK I have learned to use both. Despite miles being the preferred unit of measuring distance in the UK, there's a certain inconsistency in the units of measurement when it comes to running. We discuss our 1-mile times, but when it comes to parkrun, it's a 5k affair. We boast about our speed for a 10k, not 6.2 miles. Beyond the 10k-mark, miles tend to take over, with a half marathon measuring 13.1 miles and a marathon being 26.2 miles. Yet during a half marathon or marathon event, you might encounter kilometre countdowns! It's so confusing for beginner runners. After lots of back and forth, when it came to this book, I finally settled on using units that are in line with the UK running community, which roughly translates to kilometres up to 10k and miles thereafter. To alleviate any confusion, I've included a handy kilometre vs miles table and vice versa in my appendices and I occasionally state the equivalent distance in brackets where relevant in the book.

If you encounter any unfamiliar terms or concepts, there's a glossary waiting for you at the end of the book.

Wishing you joy in both reading and running,

Merili

Prologue

Two hours into the ultra marathon and I was already feeling tired. *How will I be able to keep going for another six?* My mind was playing tricks on me, and doubts started to creep in. However, despite being warned not to try anything new during a race, I'd packed some dried mango at the last minute. I was glad I did! When I took a bite, the sweet taste and energy it provided instantly lifted my spirits and gave me a new burst of strength. I realised that sometimes taking a risk can pay off in unexpected ways. With newfound determination, I pressed on, confident that I could overcome any obstacle the race might throw my way. I could do this!

Regardless of the fact I'd already completed two marathons before entering this ultra marathon, in the midst of actually running it I found myself struggling with doubts and self-criticism. When I caught myself walking before I'd even completed the full marathon distance, I berated myself for not sticking to my plan to run the entire distance. As a running coach, I knew the importance of walking and recovering during long races, but it was hard to take my own advice. I still struggled to see myself as a 'real' runner. However, I reminded myself that every step, whether a run or a walk, was a step towards the finish line. And in the end, that was all that mattered.

I had promised my husband I'd send updates, but my phone was not cooperating; I had never thought about the possibility of losing my phone reception during the race. Despite the frustration, I continued to type in short messages, hoping they would eventually reach him: '11.8 miles, no reception', '14.2 miles, struggling', 'feeling better, but out of water', '19.7 miles, aid station at 23 miles', '23.3 miles', '26.4 miles'. It was not just for him: seeing these messages on my phone screen gave me a sense of accomplishment and progress, which I desperately needed right then. I assumed my tracking was not working, leaving my husband clueless about my whereabouts. But these messages were my lifeline at the time, and I kept sending them every few miles.

Occasionally during the race, I encountered other runners. Some sped past me, while others I passed. But ultimately, each person had their own unique race to run, and I reminded myself to stay focused on my journey.

I struggled more than I thought I would. Running in the thick woods was peaceful, but it was also lonely. As someone who usually loved running alone, the loneliness and sense of isolation came as a surprise to me. To take my mind off the isolation I was feeling, I decided to focus on my senses. The ground was spongy under my feet, and the sound of my breathing echoed through the trees. I wished I had woods like this near my home. The temperature was perfect for running, and the smell of pine and earth filled my nose. I followed the tape and arrows that marked the route, and it felt like I knew where I was going.

Seeing other runners on the course helped me feel connected and reminded me that we were all doing this together. Sometimes I found myself running alongside others, but I was most comfortable when I could run at my own pace. Matching someone else's speed could be challenging for me, and I often ended up trailing behind. However, I did not let that discourage me. Instead, I kept pushing until I caught up.

As I approached the marathon distance, I spotted the girls I had run with earlier in the race, who were also tackling their first ultra marathon. We reached the marathon distance together and then ran together for a bit longer, but I had to let them go. It was nice to chat with them, and it made me feel less lonely. I finished the marathon distance in less than five hours, which wasn't bad considering how I was feeling. I just had to keep going.

I wondered if Lime Tree Avenue was ahead as I followed another runner and ran on the tarmac towards Clumber Park. We had passed each other a few times before. I knew the promised lime trees and the long avenue couldn't be far. Just as I got into a comfortable running rhythm, another runner shouted that I was going the wrong way. After running over 27 miles, extra mileage was not what I wanted. When I finally returned to the correct route, I passed a group of teenagers on a walking tour. I don't know how I missed the turning. My thighs were in pain, but I felt embarrassed to walk in front of the group. I told myself, *You're a runner, not a walker!* and pushed on, even though my running pace was slow.

When I finally reached Lime Tree Avenue, I was disappointed to find it empty. I had hoped to see some supporters, but there was no one there – just an endless row of lime trees. Mind you, the green leaves of the trees provided shade from the sun, and a gentle breeze rustled through them, creating a soothing sound. The sound of my footsteps echoed against the trees, and the silence around them felt almost eerie. The avenue seemed to stretch out endlessly, with no end in sight.

I tried to run, but walking seemed much nicer. I got stuck behind a tall man who was walking. He used running poles and I wondered how much they actually help. *I ought to try these*, I thought. I had overtaken him earlier in the race, but the avenue just kept going. I didn't bother to try and run past him again, so I just kept walking. I felt annoyed that he was walking, seemingly giving me ideas that walking was the better option. While I walked, I took in my surroundings and the beauty of the trees, making me appreciate the peacefulness and serenity of the moment. I told myself I would walk for a bit and then start running again. I was planning to use a 4-minute running and 1-minute walking interval. But when I tried to start running again, I wished I hadn't stopped. My legs felt like a couple of sticks attached to my body. I didn't think I could switch to running. I walked again. It just felt so much better. Who cared what my time would be? I just wanted to get to the finish line.

But deep down, I *did* still care about my time. I really wanted to finish the 40.8 miles in less than 8 hours. I pushed myself to run and promised to take shorter walking breaks to prevent feeling too stiff. As the avenue ended, my Garmin watch showed 31 miles. I was aware that technically anything beyond a marathon distance qualified as an ultra, but in the world of ultra races, the starting point was typically 31 miles. I knew I still had a long way to go, but I took comfort in the fact that I had already attained so much at this stage of the run.

After setting off for my first run on a sunny April day during the Covid-19 lockdown – two years and five weeks ago – I had become an ultra runner!

PART I:
ZERO TO MARATHON

Chapter 1:
That First Run

*You don't have to be great to start,
but you have to start to be great.*

Zig Ziglar

Where are those running shoes? I asked myself. The last time I laced up was quite a while ago now. When I first moved to England over five years ago I ran a few times, but after that I never laced up again. I'm not sure why. I think the core reason was that I found it hard and uncomfortable. Everyone seemed to be looking at me and silently judging my red face and running style. I recognised the behaviour so common for me: if I can't do it well enough (by my standards) I don't do it at all. Won't even try. Nope.

 Then Covid-19 came around, and suddenly we were all in lockdown, unable to go out when we wanted. I didn't really want to write about Covid-19 in this book, but I feel I need to. Hopefully, by the time this book is printed, Covid-19 is a distant memory for all of us. During the first lockdown, our daily routines underwent a significant change, and it felt as though our freedom had been taken away from us. It was like being imprisoned in our own home, with no visiting hours to break the monotony.

Ultimately, the pandemic and subsequent lockdowns changed how we engaged in leisure activities and exercise. Personally, I am grateful for the lockdowns that took place during the pandemic. They gave me the opportunity to discover my love for running, which has brought me so much joy and personal growth.

On the face of it, the UK Covid-19 regulations which restricted outdoor exercise to once a day may not seem like a big deal, but its impact was widespread. Seasoned runners, who were used to training with a group, participating in races, and hitting the trails on a regular basis, found themselves facing new challenges. With gyms and running tracks closed and races cancelled, many runners had to adapt to a new way of training. The lack of structure and motivation was a challenge for many, but some embraced it as an opportunity to try new forms of exercise, such as yoga or strength training. People also got more creative and ran marathons in their gardens or around their houses. I applaud all those who had the patience to do such extraordinary things.

The rise of virtual races provided runners with a new way to stay active and participate in races while following social distancing guidelines. Runners could participate in races from the safety of their own homes and neighbourhoods and still get a sense of accomplishment and community. This was an excellent option for those who wanted to stay active while in-person races were cancelled or brought a general sense of trepidation. Ultimately, the events of the past few years have shown us the importance of being able to adapt and find new ways to engage in the activities we love.

On the flip side, while the pandemic posed challenges for experienced runners, it also encouraged many new runners to take up the sport. With gyms and other indoor exercise facilities closed, people were forced to find alternative ways to stay active. Running, being a low-cost and easily accessible form of exercise, was an attractive option for many. Many of my friends used the lockdown as an opportunity to establish new exercise routines. Occasional runners became regular runners, and many of them started to do home workouts to manage the monotony of the days. Whilst children were being homeschooled, the lack of a school run and daily commute released some extra time for exercise.

For some, this was an opportunity to take up a new hobby, while for others, it was a way to cope with the stress and uncertainty of the pandemic. Additionally, with lockdowns limiting social interactions, many people turned to running to improve their mental health and relieve stress. This was definitely the case with me. Without the push from the lockdown, I don't think I would have been able to silence my self-doubting inner gremlins who, at previous attempts with running, had always tried to convince me I wasn't a runner. What was so different this time around?

At first, I was coping quite well with the lockdown. It just seemed like one of those weeks when we didn't go out much.

The weather was lovely, and my young son and I spent much time in the garden. However, homeschooling generated an additional challenge to parents who suddenly had to take on the role of a teacher. Toddler groups, which we loved to go to, went online, and my toddler wasn't having any of it. I just couldn't get him to engage with online sessions. After many unsuccessful tries, I just gave up on them. As the weeks passed, I found that being at home became more challenging. Some days were incredibly tough, as I tried to keep him occupied and make sense of it all for him. I felt trapped in my own home.

I recalled a book my mum gifted me years ago, focusing on stress relief without medication; I'd read it during my early twenties, when I was struggling with depression. Buying books is my mum's way to show she cares. Often, when she didn't know what to say to me, she would offer a book on the subject. I vividly remember a narrative from that particular book, David Servan-Schreiber's *Instinct to Heal,* about a girl named Xaviera. She had been battling depression for two years but was hesitant about therapy or medication. Despite her reservations, she agreed to participate in a study that involved running for 20–30 minutes, three times a week. After just a few runs, she began to feel less depressed, and over the following weeks, her mood continued to improve.

I remember reading this story in my bedroom in a little wooden house in one of the greenest areas in the capital of Estonia in Tallinn, Nõmme. I was studying to be an accountant at the time. When I initially read this story, I wanted to start running, but I never did. In the back of my head, I had this knowledge that running would help with mental health, but the belief that running is uncomfortable always won. The story was only a few pages long, and I couldn't recall anything else from the book, yet, for some reason, this particular story stuck with me. Now, inexplicably, I found myself recollecting the story once again.

One cold April day, I felt especially fed up with everything. Parenting is hard on a good day, but lockdown added another layer. My husband, Paul, who was working from home, used his lunch break to take over entertaining our son to give me a bit of breathing space and said, 'Go for a run.' It seemed like a strange suggestion, considering I hadn't run properly for years and have never been a runner. However, by this point I had been flirting with the idea of running for a few weeks. In that moment, getting out of the house seemed like such a good option, and, rather spontaneously, I just went.

I didn't care what everybody would think of me running. (And I thought that there wouldn't be many people out anyway.) I laced up my old leather Nike running shoes. They felt uncomfortable, but they were my only pair of trainers I owned. I wish when I'd bought them, I would have actually known something about running, and had chosen a better pair. I never really got on with that pair. When I chose them, all I was interested in was how they looked, what colour they were; functionality wasn't so important. At that period of my life, everything had to be black, including running shoes.

There I was with my uncomfortable running shoes, Lidl cotton leggings, and a hoodie. I looked nothing like a runner with my mismatching and random gear. The sun was shining brightly, and despite the lingering chill in the air, I revelled in the refreshing combination of the cold breeze and the warm sun on my face. I set off. *Here we go. It feels hard. Very hard. Let's just keep going. I will see where that road goes,* I said to myself. At that point, I had been living in our village for a good five years and I'd never actually been to the end of our road by foot. Silly, right? I had no idea how far the country lane would take me.

Years ago, I still lacked confidence behind the wheel, even after passing my driving test. I had a distant memory of driving to the end of this road to practise my driving. It seemed quite a short distance, but we all know that distance seems a lot shorter when you are driving!

My grey leggings weren't ideally suited for running; they kept slipping down. I adjusted them a few times, but eventually I decided to let them be. As long as they were covering what needed to be covered, I was okay with it. I thought I could run to the end of the road. I carried on running. The sun was out, and there were also many walkers. I didn't expect so many people to be out and about. After all, we were in lockdown. I knew that my face always turned bright red when I ran. I tried brushing off the feeling that people were judging me and laughing at my running. Somehow, I managed to keep my inner gremlins at bay and kept on running.

I ran towards the next house and then the next one. I live in the countryside, so the houses are far from each other on country lanes. Could I get to the end of the next road, or should I turn back? I was tired out already. I didn't use anything for tracking my run, but my prehistoric watch showed my steps. I tried to guess how far I had come.

I felt the urge to stop immediately rather than get to the end of the road. I decided to run to the next tree – just before the road turned a bit – and then turn around. I just wanted to have some sort of tangible landmark so that if I went for a run again I would know how far I'd been.

As part of our UK lockdown 1-hour-per-day exercise allowance, nearly every day my husband, son, dog, and I went to the nearby riverbank for a walk and some fresh air, giving our dog, Stanley, a chance to run about and spend some outside time together as a family. For nearly a month, the only place I'd been outside our house and garden was the riverbank. It was weird to see other people during my run. It felt good to be out, but at the same time, it felt awkward.

Be sensible, I reminded myself. I made it to the tree before the road took a turn, and I turned around. I didn't manage to reach the end of the lane, but that was okay. Now all I had to do was run back home. As I turned around, everything got a tiny bit easier. Knowing that half of the distance was already covered helped. Now when I run towards home it usually feels great, but it felt incredibly difficult that first time. I wanted to give up many times. To fight the desire to stop, I started to set small goals. I would just run to the next house; then to the next tree. It helped me focus on something smaller than the overall distance, making the rest of the run manageable.

Before I knew it, I was back home. Exhausted and with shaky legs, I felt proud of myself for pushing through and completing the task. I had run. I was surprised at how good it felt. I had achieved something, something that I didn't think I could do. Later, when I mapped out the run, I worked out I'd run about 4k. I felt a sense of accomplishment and pride. I couldn't wait to lace up my shoes and do it again.

Against the odds, I ventured out for a second, third, and fourth run over the next few weeks. Five months later, I completed my first marathon. Ever since that first run in my completely inappropriate trainers, I've continued running and loving it. Running is not merely an activity I endure or do because I should exercise. It has become an incredibly important part of my life, even when things don't go as planned. I'm going to share what I've learned about running in the hope that you can learn from my mistakes but also so you believe that you can do it too. You can run, whether you choose marathons or stick to 5ks. I'm going to show you all that running has to offer and how it changed me for the better.

Chapter 2:
My First Running Experiences and First Races

The journey of a thousand miles begins with a single step.

Lao Tzu

I was born and raised in Estonia, a country that has undergone significant transformation over the years. When I was a child, Estonia was still a part of the Soviet Union, and the country was experiencing a challenging period of change and upheaval. Despite this, I have fond memories of growing up in Estonia and have seen first-hand how the country has evolved into a modern, high-tech European nation.

In my early thirties, I made the decision to move to England, a country that has been my home for many years now. This move was both exciting and challenging, as I had to adapt to a new culture and navigate a different way of life. However, I have since settled in and love England and all it offers.

As a child, I was a shy girl, often hiding away and lacking in confidence. I looked up to my older sister, who exuded confidence at school, excelled in crafts, and fearlessly tried new things. I yearned to be more like her, but it just wasn't in my nature. I aspired to achieve the same high grades as her and to have as many friends as she did. I simply wished to be more like her, but I couldn't escape the fact that I was, and am, myself.

As a child, I was never particularly athletic. Between the ages of nine and eleven I was frequently absent due to illness, which meant missing school and PE classes. In hindsight, I think being bullied at school made me want to avoid school and PE, and also contributed to some serious illnesses such as pneumonia.

When I did attend PE classes, I often felt helpless. I was consistently one of the last ones chosen for team sports. I felt especially bad when PE was together with the boys. I was the target of a lot of name-calling and bullying at break times, which fuelled a constant fear of being judged and not wanting to do anything that could incite more name-calling. During one PE session we played dodgeball (a game I absolutely hated). Somehow, while attempting to catch a ball, I ended up breaking a bone in my finger. Instead of feeling sad about the impending cast, I felt relieved as it offered me a break from PE for a few weeks.

Despite my dislike for PE, I stuck with it and did what was necessary to get by, but due to missing a lot of PE classes, I found it hard to get good grades (hence the C grade). The strict norms and criteria children were expected to meet made it challenging to succeed, and falling short of these expectations was discouraging. It's not uncommon for children to feel like they are not good enough if they don't meet athletic expectations.

However, it's important to remember that every child is unique, with different abilities, interests, and strengths. It's impossible for everyone to meet the same athletic levels, and that's okay. Instead of focusing solely on these norms, it's important to encourage children to find physical activities that they enjoy and feel good doing. This can help them develop a positive relationship with physical activity and promote a lifetime of health and wellness. This is something that I certainly missed out on. I hope my son will never have to fear that he's not good enough or face bullying.

When I was a bit older (around thirteen years old), my sister and I started attending aerobics classes, and sometimes we would walk home after a session instead of taking the bus. It was a long way, but it helped ignite my love for walking – an activity I have since enjoyed throughout my life. To mix it up, my sister and I would also go for short runs, usually just for a few miles, but it was never for the joy of running. It was always with the intention of losing weight. Despite not seeing immediate results with weight loss, those runs gave me a taste for running, and I enjoyed spending time with my sister and being outside in good weather. I struggled to keep up with my sister, who was more athletic and taller, but I liked running nonetheless. *Longer legs will get you better results,* I thought at the time.

One day after school, I decided to run on my own, covering the same loop my sister and I usually ran. Running on my own, I could adjust to a pace I felt comfortable with, and I ended up running four loops, totalling around 8k, which was a significant distance for someone who was not experienced in running. I still remember the feeling I had after I'd finished that run. This was the first time I'd experienced a 'runner's high'. After completing this run, I noticed an increased confidence during PE classes: I was proud of myself and I felt more at ease.

At the time, my sister and I exercised in whatever shoes we had, just like many others who couldn't afford to buy specialist footwear. Even if you had the means to afford it, there was nothing available to purchase. It was the post-Soviet era, and the remnants of the Soviet deficit continued to shape our lives. While running wasn't a significant part of my childhood, the little bit I did taught me to appreciate the value of hard work, determination, and resourcefulness. These values have stayed with me and served me well throughout my life.

When I started high school – which in Estonia starts at age fourteen – I became increasingly concerned about my weight. In my second year of high school, I decided to try running again to lose weight. I remember getting up early and running a few times around our block of houses. It made me feel good, but sleeping longer in the mornings seemed more appealing and the original goal to lose weight never materialised. Looking back, if I had known then how much running can positively impact mental health, I might have continued with it. I've had other brief bursts of running throughout my life, but it always felt like a chore. I now realise that my mindset was a significant factor. If I had approached running with a more positive attitude and focused on the benefits beyond weight loss, I might have enjoyed it more.

Years passed, and I rarely found myself running, except for the occasional sprint to catch a bus. However, I have always enjoyed long walks, whether alone or with friends. Whenever possible, I prefer walking to taking the bus or other forms of transportation. There's something about the simplicity and freedom of walking that I find deeply satisfying. It allows me to clear my mind, connect with nature, and appreciate the world around me at a slower pace. Whether I'm exploring a new city or wandering through a familiar neighbourhood, walking has always been a reliable source of exercise, relaxation, and inspiration for me. While walking isn't the same as running, it provides an excellent foundation for building up to running. Both activities share the same goal of spending time outdoors, which can immensely benefit mental and physical well-being.

Running is a popular sport in Estonia, with numerous mapped routes available for running and walking enthusiasts alike. One of the reasons running is so popular in Estonia is due to the abundance of mass events that occur throughout the year. From marathons to charity runs, there are plenty of opportunities to participate in organised runs and connect with other runners in the community. Many workplaces also support entries for these events, recognising the physical and mental health benefits of running and walking.

Whilst I entered a few races when I lived in Estonia, I never trained seriously for them. The first race I ever participated in was when I was twenty-eight years old: a 10k event with over 6,000 runners and walkers. I remember going off too fast and suffering with stitch throughout the race, but I also recall feeling a sense of satisfaction and pride when I finally crossed the finish line.

After that initial race, I didn't enter another one for two years. I only decided to enter another one after being encouraged by my workplace. For my second race I chose to enter a 7k women-only event, and to my surprise, I found I could run the entire way without stopping. Yet again, I remember that feeling of incredible pride and attainment when I crossed the finish line, knowing that I had pushed myself to new limits and achieved something that I once thought was impossible. The following year, I decided to rerun the same race, and I was proud to improve my time by 5 minutes. I didn't see myself as a runner, though.

After those races, I got caught up in everyday life and gradually forgot about running. Occasionally, I would go out for a sporadic run and enjoy the experience, but I never kept up with it consistently. Looking back, I wonder if having someone to hold me accountable would have helped me stay more committed to running. I had friends who were runners, and sometimes they invited me to run with them. However, I nearly always declined, feeling like I probably couldn't keep up with them. I didn't want to disappoint myself or them, and it was easier to avoid the possibility of failure by not trying at all. In hindsight, I understand that my fear of failure was holding me back from truly enjoying the sport and reaping the benefits of regular exercise.

After taking an intentional break from running, I experimented with other forms of exercise and even became a regular at the gym. But I found myself enjoying those activities less than I had hoped. I was always worried about what other people thought of me and how I looked when exercising. My inner gremlins were too convincing. It took me many years to return to running and discover my true passion. Looking back, it's clear that running was always a part of me, even if I didn't realise it at the time.

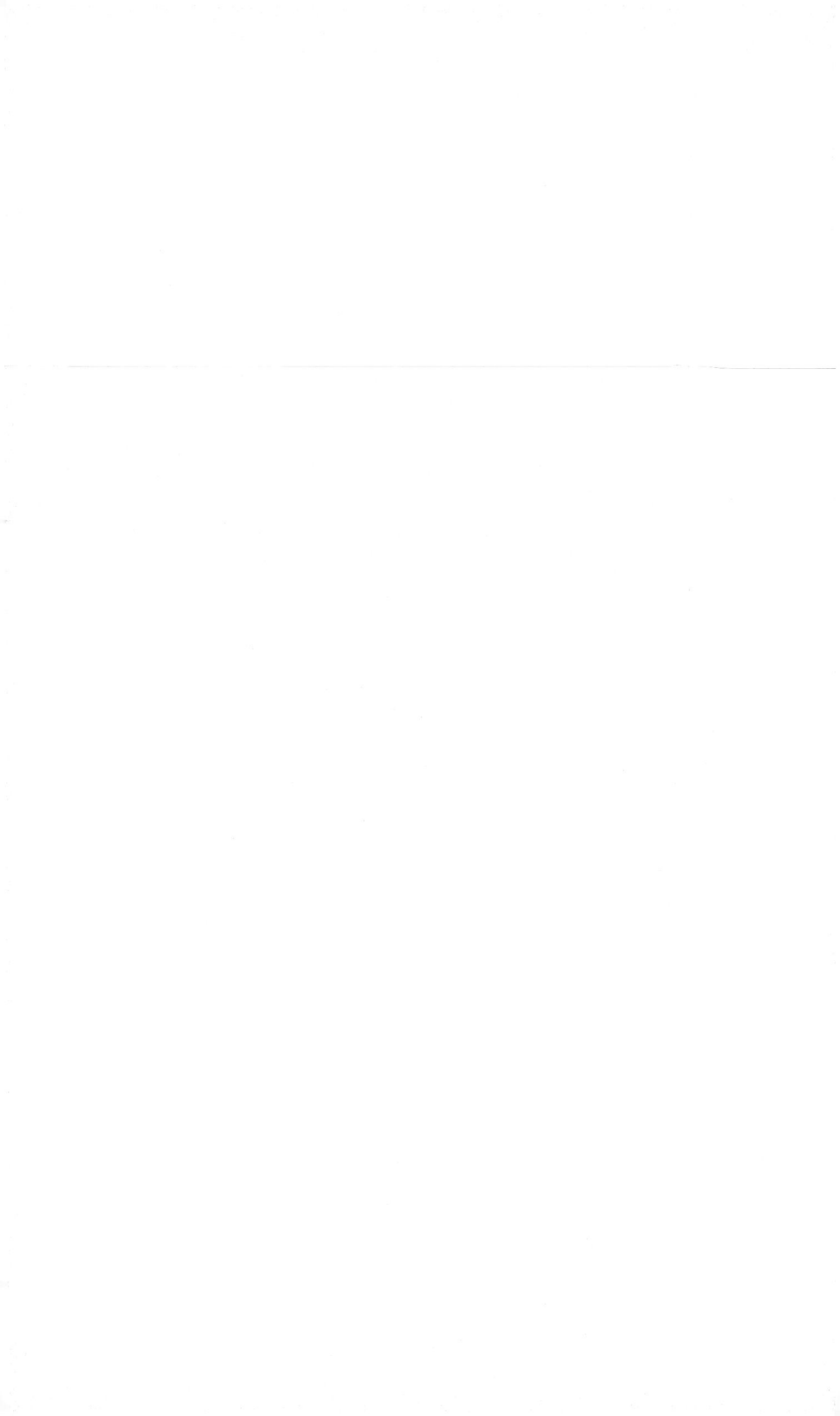

Chapter 3:
Just Run

Go as long as you can, and then take another step.

UNKNOWN

When I run, I have a personal mantra that I repeat to myself: 'just run'. To me, it means letting go of any worries about pace or other distractions and simply focusing on the joy of running. Running without constantly checking my watch or worrying about numbers is liberating and allows me to fully embrace the experience without any interruptions. I've found that my running form is also better when I'm not fixated on my watch.

When I first started running, I had yet to learn of different paces, and the only metric I focused on was distance. Looking back, I realise that it was the freedom and sense of gratification that made those early runs so special. These days, I try to recapture that feeling of unbridled joy and liberation whenever I can, even if it means temporarily letting go of my usual pace-focused mindset.

As a stay-at-home mum, when England's first lockdown began, I tried hard to provide engaging activities for my toddler. However, by the end of most evenings, I found myself exhausted. The riverbank we visited as a part of our 1-hour exercise allowance was 2.5 miles away from our home – in a different direction to where I preferred to run in those early running days. We'd drive down in our campervan (because the road was too bumpy for my little car), but more often than not my son was so upset and confused by what was going on that he refused to walk, so most of the time he and I would only walk 200–300 metres before turning back to the campervan. At least my husband and dog got a bit of a walk before he had to return to his desk in our bedroom, preparing to tackle once again the daily grind of working from home.

In the evenings, my husband and I began practising yoga together. While he loved it, I wasn't particularly motivated to do it. My mind was constantly checking the clock, waiting for the session to end so I could unwind with a glass of wine before it all started again the next day. Hurrah for wine! (I'm sure alcohol sales skyrocketed during that first lockdown.)

As much as I love my son and spending time with him, I eagerly looked forward to the weekends when my husband would be there to spend time with us. It was a welcome change to have some company and share the parenting responsibilities. Our once-a-day exercise routine during the weekends was also more relaxed as we didn't have to hurry back because of my husband's work.

My inspiration to start running came from an unexpected source: my mother-in-law. She walked 10,000 steps in her long and narrow garden every morning, and I was impressed by her dedication. At the same time, I was barely doing 3,000 steps a day. I really wanted to change that. I felt tired, unfit, and unhealthy. To stay active, I started running circles in our small garden with a goal of reaching 5,000 steps each day. Sometimes I added a few minutes of running indoors on the spot; other times I ran for short intervals in the garden while my son watched cartoons.

When I began those small running bursts, I had to admit that I had a problem. After giving birth, I started to experience stress incontinence, which never improved. Even just running after my son in the playground would cause leakage. The first few times it happened, I was incredibly upset and immediately turned to Google to find a solution. I diligently performed Kegel exercises in an attempt to improve the situation, but to no avail. In the end, I simply accepted that I had a problem that wouldn't magically disappear and opted to wear a pad during my runs.

After a few weeks of consistent effort with these garden loops, I noticed a significant improvement in my fitness level and although I was still worried people might notice any leaking, my desire to get out and do something for myself was bigger than my fear about what people thought. Paul's offer to go running came at the exact right time.

After completing my first 'proper' run, a range of questions came to mind. I knew right away that I wanted to do it again. It was a great excuse to get out and explore different scenery. But I had many questions at that point: Should I run every day or every other day? What distance should I aim for? What should I wear? Do I need to stretch? Before, after, or both? (For answers to those questions, see chapter 33.) Despite my doubts, I was determined to stick to a running routine and not give up after a few attempts, as I had done in the past (in my twenties, I had even run as far as 10 miles, but running consistently just never stuck.)

The second time I laced up I went a bit further, but still didn't manage to get to the end of the road. I didn't take note of how fast I was at that point, all I wanted to do was to keep going. When I turned back this time, I had to run uphill. I still often run this same route, and now I quite like that little hill. However, that first time felt so tough. Getting to the top without walking gave me the determination to keep running. I did what I had done the first time: I set myself those seemingly inconsequential landmarks. *Run to the next house*, I said to myself. When I got there, I focused on running to the next one. When I ran out of houses, I focused on trees, gates, or footpaths; whatever offered some goal. As I got closer to home, the distance between my 'landmarks' got shorter, but I didn't care. I was running! I think this is a valuable lesson. Just run the section you are in, even if that means focusing on a 100-metre stretch.

Those first runs in lockdown compared to running in my twenties changed my attitude towards exercise. There was something about running outside, feeling the sun, the wind on my skin, and being surrounded by nature that I found invigorating. I cleaned up an old bike and started cycling a few times a week to complement my running routine. My cycling sessions on this vintage bicycle brought back memories of my childhood when my friends and I would ride, relishing the freedom it provided. In lockdown, it also allowed me to explore potential running routes.

Additionally, I gave yoga another chance and started incorporating yoga sessions for runners into my training. This time, I found myself not impatiently waiting for the session to end so I could have some wine; instead, I genuinely enjoyed it. Before long, I was running three times a week, with the occasional bike ride in-between. I had formed a habit of exercising.

Within a few weeks, even if I had already spent my 1 hour of exercise walking on the riverbank with my family, I would feel a strong desire to go for a run. It was an unusual feeling as we had always adhered to the 1-hour exercise rule together, making sure Stanley also got some exercise. However, being alone brought a sense of freedom. For once, I didn't have anyone repeatedly calling out 'Mummy, Mummy' – as had become the norm. It was just me, responsible only for myself and my body, with the simple goal of moving forward.

Chapter 4:
I'm a Runner!

If you run, you are a runner. It doesn't matter how fast or how far. It doesn't matter if today is your first day or if you've been running for twenty years. There is no test to pass, no license to earn, no membership card to get. You just run.

JOHN 'THE PENGUIN' BINGHAM

This quote by 'the Penguin' perfectly sums up that running isn't about being fast or having a certain level of skill: it's just about putting one foot in front of the other. But for a long time, I thought that running was more complicated than that. I always thought that to be a 'proper runner' you must do extraordinary things and be someone special. I couldn't put my finger on what that something special was, but I thought that whatever it was, I didn't have it. It just wasn't me. I wasn't a runner. Even when I ran regularly three days a week and had completed a half marathon, I still felt I wasn't a real runner.

I thought that to be considered a proper runner, you had to have certain qualities and possess the right gear, like the best running shoes and clothes. When I was younger, I didn't put much thought into what kind of shoes I wore for a run. I would just grab the nearest pair of sneakers and hit the pavement. However, as I got older and I entered a few races to run with my co-workers, I invested in a pair of Nike running shoes. I chose them based on their appearance rather than comfort, and as a result, they were never truly comfortable to run in.

It wasn't until my lockdown runs that I realised just how important good gear was. When I went out for those first runs, I just put on my old running shoes. Yes, the same uncomfortable leather Nike running shoes, even though they'd also become slightly too small for me.

During my first, slow run, I felt something wasn't quite right. I stopped to tie my laces a few times, trying to make them more comfortable. After that first run, I noticed my socks were drenched in sweat, and my shoes felt tight and uncomfortable. Leather running shoes with cotton socks seems a ridiculous idea for me now, but I didn't know better at the time. My husband pointed out that good socks were key, and he was right. So I bought a pair of low-cut compression socks, which made a huge difference in keeping my feet dry and blister-free.

After a couple of runs in those Nikes, I had to admit that they weren't suitable if I wanted to carry on running. Despite my best efforts, my old shoes were simply too small and uncomfortable for me to continue wearing, and I'd started to experience some knee pain. Even with a dodgy knee, I was determined not to give up on my newfound passion, so I immersed myself in resources about running and running-specific exercises. That was when I discovered the importance of wearing running shoes that are half to a full size larger than everyday shoes; there were also different lacing patterns and exercises to alleviate pain. My only goal was to hit the pavement again. After careful consideration, I ordered a new, basic pair of running shoes online that would be better suited to my needs.

When my modest new shoes arrived, I was back in action and building up my runs again. I used my research to create my own strength and conditioning programme to do after each run, though I still wasn't sure of what I was doing. I also ordered a knee support, which helped alleviate the knee pain. I thought I'd developed knee pain from pushing myself too hard, too soon. Later on, I'd learn that muscles supporting my knees would have benefitted from more time to strengthen. Couch to 5k programmes take around 8–9 weeks for a reason, as the body needs time to adapt to the new demands of running. But I ignored all that and just ran. I was fortunate enough to continue running without causing any long-term damage.

With my replacement trainers, I could run further with far less discomfort. However, although those shoes got me out running, they wore out fast. So it was evident that I needed a new pair. My husband suggested that I should get properly fitted, and he would get me a pair for my upcoming birthday at the beginning of July. I wasn't sure about getting fitted and spending around £100 for a pair of trainers. At thirty-seven years old, I felt like a worried child, not sure what the new experience would bring. But I knew I needed to get a new pair if I wanted to carry on running, so, reluctantly, I agreed.

Prior to going to the appointment, I had read Alexandra Heminsley's *Running Like a Girl*. She described her not-so-great experience at the London Marathon shop, and I was afraid my experience would be similar. After all, I wasn't a runner. It would also be the first shop I visited since the Covid-19 lockdown. I did my food shopping online, and for everything else, Amazon Prime helped out.

I searched for running shops that offered shoe fitting near me and found two shops. I read every review I could find about both of them. While both had good reviews, for some reason I was drawn towards Lincolnshire Runner. Although I was still cautious about leaving the house due to Covid-19, I decided to book an appointment for a gait analysis. It felt strange going to a shop after so many months of lockdown, but I felt safe with the appointment-only policy. Four days before my birthday I headed to my shoe fitting.

I felt anxious. The shop was in an area I had never driven in before. Despite checking my route beforehand on Google Maps and figuring out where to park, I was worried about taking a wrong turn and not finding a parking place. I arrived a bit early for my appointment and anxiously sat in the car (I'd found a parking spot right outside the shop), waiting for my appointment time. Finally, I put on my mask and headed inside.

When I entered the shop, I was greeted by the kind owner, Keith. He didn't look like a runner, but reviews declared he was very knowledgeable and knows his stuff. To my horror, there were other people in the shop getting fitted at the same time. Pressing forwards, I tried to put my anxiety behind me and accept the situation. Looking back on it now, my anxiety about Covid-19 was disproportionate, but that's how I felt at the time.

During my shoe fitting, I had to wear a mask, and I remember feeling odd running with it on. First he asked to see my current shoes. Sheepishly, I took my worn-out pair of Mountain Warehouse running shoes out of the bag. He looked at my shoes, examined their wear and asked, 'How often do you normally run?'

'I run three times a week: two shorter runs and a longer run on Sundays,' I answered, not really knowing if it was enough running to be considered a runner. He then asked me to hop on the treadmill. I clung tightly to the handrails, feeling that I couldn't run properly on it. My hands got sweaty, and my glasses steamed up as I tried to keep my cool. For a moment, I thought, *Do I really need those shoes that much to feel like this?*

Fortunately, after observing my attempt to run on a treadmill and realising it wouldn't work for me, he asked me to run outside, where he monitored my running form. I picked a lamp post in the distance and started running back and forth, feeling slow and awkward under scrutiny. Some people passed by, adding to my anxiety. I thought they must think what an idiot I was, running back and forth next to the running shop. After a few attempts, I realised I was still wearing my mask. I could have taken it off outside, but I didn't even notice it amid all my other worries.

Keith then brought out three pairs to choose between. When I started running I joined many Facebook running groups, and a lot of the runners were obsessed with Brooks. They seemed to be a runner's holy grail. I thought having Brooks running shoes would make me a real runner, the proper one. The first pair I tried was Brooks. I loved how they looked, and the colour scheme was just to my liking. As soon as I put them on, however, they felt small. We sized up. My normal shoe size is 5, but I run in a size 6. I had to try the size 6.5 for Brooks. I hoped that Brooks would be the one, and I would join all those 'real runners' sporting their beautiful running shoes. After only a few steps, however, I knew these wouldn't be the ones. I really wanted them to be, but no, I had to admit the defeat: it just wasn't a good fit for me.

The second pair I tried were Mizuno Wave Riders. I really didn't like how they looked: the colour seemed awful – a mix of light red and dark red, just ugly. They didn't appeal. When I put them on, though, they were really comfortable to run in. It felt like running on clouds, and they just felt right. After finishing my test run with that pair, Keith looked at me and asked, 'Do you get any knee pain?'

'I did to start with, but then I picked up an exercise routine to strengthen my knees, and I don't get pain any more,' I answered. 'I do single-leg squats and several other exercises to strengthen my knees,' I added, proudly.

'Keep it up, because it seems that you are managing it,' he commented. I couldn't help but feel a bit smug. I thought non-runner me, Merili, didn't know much about running, but by the sounds of it, I was getting some things right.

The last pair he wanted me to try were some lighter stability shoes, which I hated instantly. I tried to run in them and it just didn't feel right at all. He agreed that I would be better off continuing with my exercises and sticking with neutral shoes. He added that although it's a personal choice, stability shoes could cause issues in the long run if you actually don't need them.

I tried the first two pairs again, really hoping that the Brooks would somehow have become a bit more comfortable, but no. The Brooks weren't for me. It turns out I loved running with those ugly Mizunos. They seemed spot on for me. So, despite the ugly colour, I eventually settled on a pair of Mizuno Wave Riders 23s.

'Do you have any different colours for the Mizunos?' I asked Keith, feeling a bit embarrassed that the colour mattered to me so much. He checked in the back, and while I was waiting near the tills I noticed a bright yellow Lincolnshire Runner shirt. Buying a running shirt wasn't in my agenda. Back in Estonia, I'd volunteered a few times with a friend at a local marathon and always received a race shirt as a thank you from organisers. So I had some running shirts to wear, but still, the shirt caught my eye.

When Keith got back from checking the other colours, he said, 'No, it's just this one colour.'

Still trying to convince myself that the colour doesn't matter, I answered, 'I'll still take these, please.'

Then I asked about the shirt and which size he'd recommend for me. He suggested I could use it for winter running as well, over a long sleeve top. 'Yellow would make you more visible to cars.' At this point, I had no clue about winter running, and winter seemed so far away, but I decided to listen to him and convinced myself that the grey shirt next to the yellow one was just too boring.

As I was driving home, I remembered this running shirt, which read 'I'm a Lincolnshire Runner'. It was at that moment that it truly hit me: I was not just a mum and a wife, I was a runner too. The realisation filled me with excitement and pride, so much so that I missed my turn whilst lost in thought.

Looking back, that first proper pair of running shoes I ever bought will always hold a special place in my heart. They marked the beginning of my running journey, the moment when I made the conscious decision to take my fitness and health into my own hands. Though I've since retired those shoes, they still rest at the bottom of my wardrobe as a reminder of how far I've come and how much I've achieved; they symbolise my dedication and commitment to living a healthier, happier life. Through my running journey, I've discovered that being a runner doesn't necessitate running races or participating in parkruns. You can simply go for a quiet run on your own and still be a runner. And even if you decide not to run at times, that's okay too. Remember, you are still awesome, and you should feel proud of yourself.

Chapter 5:
Marathon?

Believe you can and you're halfway there.

THEODORE ROOSEVELT

Although I had been doing some exercises I'd found (with the help of Google) to strengthen my knees, some of my runs would start with knee pain, though it usually disappeared as soon as I warmed up. However, I had a nagging feeling that something wasn't quite right, and I began searching for solutions to fix the issue. That's when I came across the book *Science of Running* by Chris Napier, which I purchased to see if it contained any useful insight to help improve my running.

With the book's guidance, I self-diagnosed myself with runner's knee, a common running injury that often affects those who push themselves too hard too soon, and the condition can also be caused by muscular imbalances. To continue running without aggravating my runner's knee, I incorporated the exercises outlined in *Science of Running* into my exercise routine, combining these exercises with the programme I had already implemented when my knee pain first appeared. After each run, I diligently followed the routine to strengthen my muscles and prevent future injuries. Between runs, I religiously iced and elevated my knee. I was heartened to hear Keith confirm that what I'd picked up from Chris's book seemed to be working. I had discovered something that made me feel good, and I wasn't ready to stop.

As I made running a regular part of my life, I noticed significant progress, even though I was still very slow. I increased my distance almost every time I ran. Although I knew about the recommended 10% weekly increase in distance, I felt good and really needed the time for myself, so I exceeded far beyond the 10% increase. It was an exciting time, full of new milestones, and I felt better after every run.

Nearly three weeks had passed since my first run when I decided to go a bit further. I remember my first 8k run vividly. At the time, it seemed like such a daunting distance! I usually ran in the evenings when my son was in bed. Finding time during the day was challenging, as my husband was busy tackling the extra workload that Covid-19 brought and wasn't really able to take breaks long enough for my runs. I enjoyed running in the evenings: the country roads where I ran were quiet, it wasn't dark, and I didn't feel pressured for time. This allowed me to run slower and longer.

That day, I ran my usual route from my doorstep, which was 6.6k. As I approached the last kilometre, I felt that maybe I could do 7k instead, so I ran down the lane to reach my desired mileage. During this extra distance, I felt that I could actually go a bit longer, so I did. During that final, eighth kilometre, I felt elated. Don't get me wrong, running still felt hard, but I was so proud of myself for pushing for 8k. I couldn't wait to get home and casually drop the news to my husband that I had just completed an 8k run (although I was bursting with pride for accomplishing such a feat).

After completing that 8k run, I felt motivated to push myself further during my next run. That's when I ran a magical 10k. Although this run was nearly 15 minutes slower than my current 10k time, I was still incredibly proud of myself for running the entire distance. In my first attempt at a 10k race, over a decade ago, I was untrained and didn't know much about running. I started too fast, got stitch early on, and had to resort to walking and running to complete the race. All I can recall from that race is the stitch, the finish line, and the free banana at the end.

A decade later, this time when I ran 10k on my own and ran the whole way, I found that I was actually slower than I had been during that previous race. However, I was proud of myself for how far I had come since then, and I knew that with persistence and dedication, I would continue to improve.

I often refer to those runs during lockdown as my first runs because it was the first time I genuinely enjoyed running. In the past, the sporadic bursts of inconsistent running I had were always driven by the wrong reasons: attempting to lose weight, avoiding feeling left out at work, or just not being able to say no when invited. The few enjoyable runs I had in my twenties just didn't stick for one reason or another; running just didn't seem to be my thing. This time around, amidst the challenges of lockdown, running became a source of solace and joy. It wasn't about external expectations or societal pressures; it was a personal journey, allowing me to discover the pure pleasure of the activity itself. These runs marked a shift, where each step felt like a conscious choice for my well-being rather than a means to an external goal.

Running provided me with a sense of accomplishment that I never expected. I believe part of this was due to the fact that I was doing it on my own terms. I had no one to answer to: I could push myself when I felt capable and take it easy when I needed to. When I had tried running in the past, I constantly compared myself with runners whose pace was too fast for me. This time, my approach was different. I took control of my training and my runs, and my only goal was to surpass my own expectations. With this new mindset, I was able to find my own pace, build my endurance, and improve at my own rate. Running became a source of empowerment for me, and it gave me a sense of ownership over my physical fitness journey.

It didn't take me long to progress from running 10k to 14k and eventually a half marathon distance of 13.1 miles. In the early days of my running journey, my main focus was simply to run a little further each time. I didn't use a watch to track my pace during runs, just the Runkeeper app on my phone, but I still felt a sense of fulfilment every time I extended my distance. From then on, I made it a rule that no run should be shorter than 10k, and if it was, I would make up the remaining distance on another day. I still follow this rule when I feel fit and healthy, though during periods when my body feels run-down, I am grateful for every run, no matter how short or long. It's important to listen to your body, not just follow some rule book. Oh, and don't start as aggressively as I did! As a trained running coach, I would recommend following a proper plan and giving your body time to adjust to the increased distance. For me, the restriction of lockdown and the sense of triumph were the driving forces that pushed me, even if it was a bit foolish.

Five weeks after my first attempt at running, I accidentally ran a half marathon. It always seemed like an unattainable goal reserved only for accomplished runners, and I never thought I could achieve it. But on that particular evening, I went out for what I thought would be a 9-mile run, not realising that I would end up running half a marathon. I was embarrassed to share that goal with Paul because running even 9 miles felt like a significant feat, so I didn't want to jinx it by telling him beforehand.

I had packed some gels to test during my longer runs but removed them from my running belt just before heading out, thinking I wouldn't need them. I felt great as I began my run, using the Runkeeper app on my phone to track my progress. The evening was pleasant, although a bit windy. When I reached 9 miles, I felt like I could go the half marathon distance, so I just kept going. Despite feeling the weight in my legs and some pain in my hips, I persevered. It was a challenging experience, but I finally completed my run just before dark, feeling exhausted but elated.

After that first half marathon, the sky seemed bluer, and everything seemed possible. I began to push myself harder during my training runs, and soon enough, I started dreaming of running a marathon. The idea of running a marathon was compelling, but I wasn't quite prepared to commit to it yet. I even looked up a marathon training plan and started to follow it loosely, to see if I could learn to commit to it. No actual marathon in sight, it was just a dream that I kept to myself.

With no particular goal in mind, I kept building on my distance and nearly two months later, during one Sunday morning long run, I challenged myself to run 19 miles. It wasn't the most rational decision (it wasn't on the marathon plan I was trying out) but I was simply following my intuition at the time; just doing what felt right. During that run, my husband and son came to say hello and brought me an extra gel; Paul also took some pictures. He posted them on Facebook and wrote that I was training for a marathon. Seeing my goal in writing, shared with the public, made it feel more real and achievable. Even though I had only started running a few months earlier, my goal was now set and clear: I was training for a marathon.

Chapter 6:
Eating Sticks and Leaves

Let food be thy medicine and medicine be thy food.

HIPPOCRATES

My personal journey towards adopting healthy eating habits has been a long and difficult one. I have struggled for most of my life with a complicated relationship with food, which I believe was rooted in my childhood.

I vividly remember being the last one at the table during meals at kindergarten, where we were expected to finish everything on our plates. However, I struggled to eat some of the foods served, particularly those with meat or lumpy textures, which I found unappetising. As I got older, I eventually learned to eat meat, but I still avoid lumpy textures to this day. At home, although there were many foods I didn't particularly enjoy, I still made an effort to eat a variety of different foods.

As a child, I remember occasionally overindulging on foods I loved and feeling uncomfortably full afterwards, though I also developed a habit of keeping some special treats for another time. I have a distinct memory of having chocolates in my dress pocket, only to have my mum wash the dress and ruin the chocolates. I still remember how upset I was.

As a teenager, my sister and I were fixated on losing weight. Our mother has struggled with weight issues her whole life, and I recall her discussing the 'point values' of various foods. Although I was not overweight as a child, I lacked confidence and generally had low self-esteem. Being skinny gave me a sense of self-worth, despite knowing deep down that it wasn't not a healthy mindset to have.

During my teenage years I seemed to attract people with disordered eating into my life. Despite not really knowing what bulimia was, being around beautiful souls (as I saw them) engaging in binge-purge cycles normalised such behaviour for me. It was only later, while reading a book about Princess Diana, that I became aware of the term 'bulimia', though I still didn't fully grasp the severity of the condition at that time.

My sister and I tried various diets, including the Atkins and cabbage soup diets. In my final year of high school (age seventeen), I had a very beautiful and skinny classmate. She shared that she had been overweight in the past but had lost the weight by eating simple, healthy foods such as salads, fruits, and buckwheat. I attempted to follow the same approach, and although it was successful, it required hard work and often left me feeling hungry.

My weight dropped, and I thought I looked stunning on my graduation photos. Looking back, I understand now I wasn't very kind to my body and was starving it through the exam period. Knowing what I know now about nutrition, my diet at the time wasn't balanced, lacked protein, and I didn't consume enough calories. My experiences in my teenage years shaped my relationship with food, making healthy eating a constant struggle for me in later life, and as I grew older, I continued to be concerned about my weight.

In my late teens and twenties, I started occasionally engaging in the binge-purge cycle myself. Over the years, I struggled with this disorder on and off, causing me significant physical and emotional distress. There were times when it was really burdensome, as it influenced all aspects of my life, leaving me feeling overwhelmed by the shame I was feeling. I would put myself through periods of strict restriction which nearly always ended with overeating episodes. I still vividly remember making myself sick in a grimy dorm bathroom during my first year of university. Back then, I was on an extremely tight budget and couldn't afford to waste any food. Consequently, I indulged in inexpensive items, whatever I could afford, even though they were often far from tasty.

Somehow, I managed to put a stop to it. Reading and learning how binging and purging negatively impacts on my body was one of the things that helped. It was far from easy and didn't happen overnight, but I silenced those inner gremlins that insisted I couldn't quit. Despite the challenges, I was fortunate enough to seek help and support and gradually learned how to manage my symptoms and pursue a healthier relationship with food. I am truly grateful for the wonderful therapist I saw at the time, who helped me put things into perspective and provided the non-judgemental listening ear I needed. These days, there are times when I hardly think about it, but it still pops up from time to time.

During my upbringing and for much of my adulthood, I believed that meat and dairy were essential components of a healthy diet. Milk was especially emphasised in my childhood. Although as a child I wasn't all that keen on meat, I gradually learned to incorporate it into my diet as I grew older.

I knew a few people in the UK who followed a plant-based diet but I had very little knowledge about it. My initial interest in a plant-based diet stemmed from a desire to improve my overall eating habits. In 2016, my husband and I decided to eliminate sugar from our diet, but my pregnancy cravings proved too strong to resist. However, in 2020, we decided to make another attempt at giving up sugar and successfully stuck to our plan. Although I still experienced cravings for sweet foods, I managed to satisfy them with dried fruit and nuts.

One evening while I was running, my husband watched the documentary film *The Game Changers* and proposed switching to a plant-based diet. Although I was initially hesitant due to my lack of familiarity with this type of food and concerned about preparing meals for my family, we decided to give it a try. We began by replacing the meat in some of our favourite meals with plant-based alternatives. Over the course of the following month, we gradually eliminated meat and dairy from our diet, finding the transition to be more manageable than expected. My husband and I opted to continue feeding our son dairy, eggs, and fish, and we will leave it to him to make his own choices about his diet in the future. Currently, he consumes a significant amount of plant-based food and takes pride in sharing the vegan products he enjoys with his friends.

I made the switch to a plant-based diet in the middle of training for my first marathon. I had always experienced a runny nose while running and I read somewhere that dairy makes a runny nose worse. I was annoyed that I always needed to carry a tissue with me on my runs, so I thought it couldn't hurt to go without dairy; it was another factor that steered me to change my diet. Eliminating dairy didn't completely stop my runny nose, but it certainly reduced it.

The lockdown period made it easier for me to adopt a plant-based diet as there was no pressure from social situations. Although I have encountered negative comments from others, I have grown more resilient to them over time. Eating out has been relatively easy as most restaurants now offer vegan options on their menus – you just need to check in advance. People's perceptions of vegan food have improved as more delicious and flavourful options become available. Vegan food is no longer seen as just 'sticks and leaves' but rather as a diverse and satisfying culinary choice (when prepared the right way).

It has taken some trial and error, but through the process of going plant-based, I have discovered what works best for my body, and I make a conscious effort to listen to its needs. I prioritise consuming a variety of whole foods and aim to eat a rainbow of colours. Whether it was the shift to plant-based foods or a change in my mindset from running, I found it logical to focus on fuelling my body for running, so worrying about eating too much or too little was never a concern during my marathon training. I ate when I was hungry and aimed to give my body what it was craving. I firmly believe that making healthy food choices has contributed to my success as a runner by allowing me to run longer and faster. Transitioning to a plant-based diet has been a helpful addition to my running journey, and the shift was relatively smooth for me. I naturally shifted to cutting out caffeine, too, as I found my body seemed to function better without it.

Then there was an unexpected, more beneficial outcome from all this. For the first time in a long time, I felt great in my body. It didn't matter how my body looked: what mattered was what I could do with it. And I was able to run many happy miles. In the past, what I thought about myself was heavily dependent on the number on my scales. When it comes to running, however, the number on the scales doesn't show how good a runner you could be: it doesn't correlate with your running ability. Things changed when I realised that how skinny I am doesn't define me. This doesn't show how good or bad a person I am. Not constantly weighing myself gives the freedom not to worry about it.

My journey towards healthy eating has been a rollercoaster of ups and downs. From childhood pickiness, teenage dieting, to my adult struggles with weight and general health. Although it can be challenging at times, I have learned to tune into my body's signals and make choices that promote both physical and mental well-being. After years of trying different diets and approaches, I've finally found what works for me: a plant-based diet filled with a variety of whole foods, limited processed sugar and caffeine, and occasionally enjoying options like a plant-based burger and a glass of wine. My focus has shifted from solely focusing on weight loss to prioritising my overall health and well-being. I am mindful of my food choices and choose those that benefit my body the most.

I am grateful for the lessons I have learned and the progress I have made on my journey towards healthy eating. It's not always easy, but the reward is completely worth it, allowing me to live simply, happily, and in harmony with the earth.

Chapter 7:
Taper Turmoil

The taper is like the calm before the storm.
Embrace it, trust it, and let it do its job.

Unknown

Choosing a race for my first marathon was a complex process. Although Covid-19 restrictions were starting to lift by the time my marathon training was due to finish, I still wasn't sure if in-person races would be taking place, and I still felt anxious about Covid-19. The thought of participating in a mass event with many runners and potentially having to wear a mask during parts of it didn't appeal to me. As I had been running alone since starting in April of that year, the idea of lining up with all those seasoned runners at a big race starting line felt intimidating. It just seemed safer and easier to do it on my own, like I was used to, so I started looking for a virtual marathon.

Running solo had become a source of comfort for me, allowing me to focus solely on my own abilities and goals without any distractions or pressure from others. The thought of navigating through crowds and potential safety risks added an unnecessary layer of stress to the experience. Ultimately, participating in a virtual race provided me with the perfect compromise. I could maintain my comfort level by running alone while still being able to challenge myself. The virtual format allowed me to participate in my own way, on my own terms, and still feel a sense of connection to the larger running community.

I chose to run my first marathon on 27 September, one week before the Virtual London Marathon event. My lucky number is 7, so I wanted to have a 7 in the date. I would have liked to run the Virtual London Marathon, but the date didn't work for me. Instead, I signed up for a completely random virtual marathon that was running on 27 September, choosing it solely based on the appearance of the medal. The medal for this virtual race was a beautiful wooden medal inscribed with the phrase 'I ran it anyway. Nothing stops me.', which I felt was a fitting tribute to receive after completing my first (solo) marathon.

When I first shared my plan with some experienced runners that I would run my first marathon solo as a virtual race, I was met with some scepticism. Many advised me that it wouldn't be an easy feat to complete on my own. Despite their doubts, I remained steadfast in my belief that I could and would do it. After all, I had developed a strong love for running alone and felt confident in my abilities. Running solo had become a way for me to disconnect from the world and focus on my own goals and abilities. It was a time to clear my mind and push myself to new limits. While I appreciated the wisdom and advice from those seasoned runners, I knew that this was something I had to do on my own terms.

After making the decision to run a marathon, I found that things were going smoothly. I followed a free training plan from MarathonPal.com, which promised to get me to the finish line by only running three times a week. On my non-running days, I stayed active and focused on reaching my daily step goal. I also added strength training into my routine, three days a week.

While I didn't follow the plan to the letter, I stuck to the main principles and never skimped on distance. I found the intervals challenging but each week I aimed to complete two faster, shorter runs, with one being a tempo run. During this training I had a very basic Garmin watch that didn't allow me to set up my own intervals, meaning I relied on my phone apps for interval training. More often than not, I simply wanted to run – run freely without bothering about following the intervals precisely. Occasionally, I incorporated some fartleks and strides into my routine to mix things up and challenge myself. I loved the lack of structure in fartleks: I could run completely intuitively, but still include some speedy sections, learning how to vary my pace and intensity based on how they felt. I sometimes added strides at the end of my run, after reading about them in Chris Napier's book.[1] I found strides fun! I usually sprinted between lamp posts. Fast running for short bursts made me feel capable, free, and, in a way, gave me childlike excitement.

As I progressed through the training plan, I began to feel more confident in my abilities and saw noticeable improvements in my running. It seemed that everything was going well, and I was on track to reach my goal of running a marathon.

That's what I thought, anyway.

Remember that somewhat stupid 19-mile run I mentioned at the end of chapter 5? In my head I really wanted to run 20 miles that time, but just before the end it felt impossible to carry on running. I had an awful stitch, no energy; it just didn't feel right. I hit the wall. I had read many descriptions about runners hitting the wall during the marathon, and that 19-mile run was my one and only encounter with it so far. The run had gone really well until I suddenly felt that I simply couldn't take another step. I was less than a mile from my house but I couldn't run if my life depended on it. I sat down at the side of the road, drank some water, and started walking home. I had to stop several times, even when walking, because I just didn't have any energy. Thankfully, no one was out to see my struggles. When I made it home, I sat down, had some electrolyte drink and some food, and felt fine shortly after. I brushed the experience off as bad luck and celebrated the 19 miles I reached before I had to stop.

I continued running as usual, but this experience truly scared me and I couldn't shake off my worries. *Maybe I am not made for marathon running?* I thought. I began researching what it was that I had experienced and concluded that I had neglected the need for electrolytes during my longer runs, especially in hot conditions. In my newfound runner's bliss, I had been running with just water and gels, thinking that would be enough. Additionally, I recognised that I had got carried away and promised to follow my training plan properly from that point on, refraining from adding extra mileage when I felt like it.

For the next six weeks I followed my plan and did well. Things were looking good. Then it was time for my longest run to date – 20 miles. I was anxious, but reminded myself that I'm smarter and fitter now and this time I will reach my goal. My positive self-talk paid off as my run went better than expected and I felt on top of the world. Not only did I finish faster than planned, but I also felt great throughout the run, with no issues or stitch. The best part? I did it all on my own, carrying my supplies and pacing myself.

As I finished this 20-mile run, I felt I still had enough energy to keep going. It was a monumental moment of pride and a huge boost for my self-belief. I knew I was ready for the marathon, and I couldn't wait for race day to arrive. Just bring it on!

I was looking forward to the easier runs coming up in the taper period. I had read about tapering and learned that the taper period in the final weeks of marathon training is essential to allow the body to recover from intense training, heal any minor injuries, and restore energy levels. I wasn't expecting to find tapering to be such a challenging and emotional experience.

After my first 20-mile run, which had gone so well, every subsequent run became a struggle. During my next long run, which was 13 miles, I had a terrible experience. My heart rate was elevated, and I struggled throughout the entire run. This problematic run led to self-doubt, and I began to question if I had what it takes to complete a full marathon if I was struggling so much during a shorter distance. After this run, it felt like I couldn't even run 6 miles, let alone a full marathon. Unfortunately, the subsequent runs didn't give me much hope either, as running continued to feel incredibly challenging.

Mentally, I was unprepared for the tapering period, which drove me mad. The self-doubt ramped up as I couldn't understand why I struggled so much. I began to question whether I was overtrained and if I was fuelling my body correctly. By then, I had been following a plant-based diet for a few months and now I wondered if I was giving my body the nutrients it needed to perform at its best. These doubts only added to the mental strain I was battling.

I knew there could be challenges that come with tapering before a marathon, but I wasn't fully prepared for its impact on my mental state. Although I had heard other runners discuss experiencing pains, a lack of confidence, and other issues before a race, I never thought I would undergo the same. I felt so good about my preparation and was confident that I was ready for the marathon. Additionally, since I was running the virtual race solo from my home, I thought removing the added pressure of the logistics of the race would make it easier.

To add to my pre-race anxiety, just two weeks before my planned marathon, my son and husband fell ill with a heavy cold. Despite my best efforts to avoid getting sick, I also caught it. As I researched whether running with a cold was safe, my anxiety only increased. Nevertheless, as I felt capable, I made sure not to miss a scheduled run during this sickness period.

As the final week before the marathon approached, I started to feel a glimmer of hope. My cold symptoms had finally subsided, and I felt a surge of energy and excitement about the upcoming race. I knew that I couldn't significantly improve my physical form in that short time, so I focused on maintaining my training and taking care of myself both mentally and physically.

During my easy runs, I used the time to reflect on my journey and how far I had come. Despite the struggles of the tapering period and the doubts that had plagued me, there had also been moments of triumph and progress. I reminded myself of the reasons why I wanted to run a marathon: fulfilling a personal victory and the feeling of pushing my limits.

My last 5k run before the marathon felt like a breakthrough. I was surprised by my pace, my heart rate was lower than usual, and I noticed my VO2 max had increased to 46, a significant improvement from my initial VO2 max of 38. It was the confidence boost I needed after struggling through the tapering period. I started to believe that I could actually do this, and my anxiety started to dissipate.

In the final days leading up to the marathon, I ate healthily and stayed hydrated, avoiding any new or heavy foods that could upset my stomach. I also tried to get as much rest as possible, although my nerves and excitement made it difficult to sleep soundly. The day before the marathon, I followed the traditional carb loading routine. Looking back, I realised I should have eaten what I craved and not put so much emphasis on carbs. Following a plant-based diet meant carb loading wasn't necessary.

As the marathon day approached, I felt a mix of nerves and excitement. I had prepared as much as I could, both physically and mentally, and now it was time to put all that training and preparation to the test. The tapering period may have driven me mad, but it was all part of the journey to becoming a marathon runner. I was ready.

Chapter 8:
Part of 1%

I've learned that finishing a marathon isn't just an athletic achievement. It's a state of mind; a state of mind that says anything is possible.

JOHN HANC

I'd waited so long for that day. I was ready. Everything was meticulously prepared the night before. I checked the weather forecast hundreds of times and carefully selected gear that I felt comfortable with. My kit list had evolved alongside my running journey, thanks to the guidance from Facebook running groups, books, and Google. Since I primarily ran alone, I had numerous opportunities to practise and determine what worked best for me.

Equipped with my hydration vest, water bladder, gels, and salt tablets, I felt ready. In many ways, it was the same as my usual Sunday morning long run. The only difference was that I had more gels in my hydration vest than usual, and I had packed a bag for my husband (who would be checking in on me along the route) with 'just in case' items.

I was eager to get out and start running. I'd slept reasonably well the night before; I woke up early and went through my usual pre-run routine, including applying nappy cream to my toes to prevent blisters, and any other areas that might rub and cause discomfort. I even retrieved a bottle of prosecco from the depths of the utility room cupboard and placed it in the fridge, ready for whatever the outcome of the race may bring. Regardless of the final result, I knew I would celebrate with a glass.

Before I set off, my son Jacob had woken up and said his usual, 'Mummy, have a good run.'

As I started my run, Paul took a few photos of me heading out. To ensure I didn't fall short of the marathon distance, I walked to the village before starting my run. Even though I had measured the marathon distance on the map, I couldn't completely trust it. I didn't want to have to run past my house to finish the race. I thought that running towards home at the end of the race would help keep me motivated. (The importance of the finish line wouldn't be a concern in an in-person race, as the finish line would be a set location.)

I decided to run my first marathon on the route I had used for most of my training runs. I wasn't very creative with my route: I wanted it to be on quiet roads with non-existent traffic. This decision had its flaws. It wasn't really a loop: I had to run to the end of one road and back, followed by running to the end of another road and then repeat that whole route three times in total to cover the distance. Despite its monotony, this route was my comfort zone; I knew it so well.

I started off in good spirits and at a good pace. Everything was going according to plan. When I ran past our house for the first time, I thought that maybe capris would have been a better choice of clothing instead of long leggings, but I didn't want to change and start again, so I told myself I was okay with my clothing choice.

My training runs leading up to the race had focused on getting my running heart rate low, and as my training progressed I was pleased to see that my efforts had paid off as my heart rate while running had decreased since I first started running. During my previous long runs, I mostly managed to keep my heart rate on the lower side.

Well, not this time. My heart rate was relatively high from the start and peaked even higher around one hour in. I didn't know what to do. I had severe self-doubt. I didn't know how I was able to do this when I felt so crap so early on. My mind was racing with negative thoughts like *You can't do this, your runs have been crap for the past few weeks; what were you expecting?* I tried to challenge my thoughts. *You can do this! You have worked really hard. Just keep going; it will get better, it always does.*

As I was approaching the river the wind felt brutal. I had run in windy weather before, but only for a short time. This time the wind felt cold; the road lonely and repetitive. The air, thick with the scent of earth and upcoming autumn, seemed to resist each stride, demanding a heightened effort from every muscle. The gusts whipped across the open landscape, tugging at the hood of my grey top and tousling my hair. I tried to use my hood to give me a bit more protection from the wind. It felt unforgivingly bitter. I sure was glad I hadn't changed into those capris!

Despite this elemental struggle, I felt exhilaration; a feeling of being alive and running my first marathon. Yet at the same time worry crept in. *It shouldn't be so hard,* I was thinking, finding it impossible to remain my pace. *After this round, I have to come here another two times today.* As the riverbank stretch came to an end, I felt relieved as the wind seemingly eased a bit, but I was still struggling to calm down my mind and ease my worry about what lied ahead.

As I was reaching 8 miles I called my husband: he is my rock and I just didn't know what else to do. He didn't answer right away, but called me back. I spluttered down the phone, 'Dear, I am really struggling. It's really windy and my watch shows that my heart rate is in the 190s. I am not sure I can do this. Could you come in the car and give me a bit of pep talk, please?'

He told me he'd come and find me, and I kept running. Even though the virtual marathon format allowed for breaks or doing it another day, I wanted it to be as close to the real thing as possible. If there was a break then my time would reflect that. I was mostly confused and frustrated about why my heart rate was so high, especially after all my training. I tried to reassure myself that my watch's heart rate monitor might not be accurate.

As I kept running, Paul eventually caught up with me in the car. He was concerned about my high heart rate and urged me to stop running.

'How do I sound?' I asked him, breathing heavily, but able to form a complete sentence without feeling I was going to die.

'You sound okay to me,' he replied, 'but how about if I stick with you for the next few miles?' His reassurance put my mind at ease, and I reasoned with myself that if my heart rate was indeed that high, I wouldn't be able to speak in complete sentences. He drove a few hundred metres ahead, waited for me, then drove ahead again, repeating this process for the next 3 miles.

Gradually, my heart rate started to drop to a manageable level. At this point, my only goal was to finish the race in under 5 hours, which was my most conservative goal. As I continued, the miles seemed to stretch out endlessly, and the route became monotonous. Despite having run these same roads many times before, this time they felt tedious. The second time I approached the riverbank, I knew what to expect. I knew it would be hard. The wind, though formidable, became a companion in my journey, pushing me to dig deeper and find strength within. I had to keep reminding myself of why I was doing it. I kept going, but it was a struggle.

My friend Irene, who had recently completed an Ironman in my hometown of Tallinn, was about to join me virtually for my final 9 miles. That provided me with a lot of motivation, as I didn't want to disappoint her. Although we weren't running together physically and weren't even in contact via phone, just knowing that she was running simultaneously with me was so uplifting. The idea that someone as amazing as she was participating in this virtual marathon with me brought me a great sense of comfort.

During the second part of my marathon I found myself waiting for her to join. In the rhythm of my strides, I could almost feel Irene's presence, a silent partner in the last stretch of the marathon. As each mile unfolded, I drew strength from the shared virtual space we occupied, finding solace in the knowledge that Irene, with her indomitable spirit, was navigating her own path at the same time. Her silent camaraderie spurred me onward, reinforcing the belief that, even in the solitude of this marathon, the support of a friend could be felt in every step.

Paul was amazing. He put aside everything to support and help me finish my marathon. Due to the early start of my race and my reliance on his support, even our dog missed his morning walk that day. I needed my husband's help so much that I'd hesitated to continue without him when he told me he needed to head off to walk the dog.

When I ran over 20 miles, I was so proud of myself for surpassing that distance. My body felt even heavier and started to hurt, but I said to myself, *I can and I will finish this run.* Now that I'd gone past the 20 miles, I could count back my last 10k (6.2 miles). During long runs, I always counted back the last 10k. Somehow, mentally, it makes it easier. It's like, *Come on, Merili, you can run another 10k. You have done it so many times before … Just 7k to go!* Once it gets to 5k, the distance left to run just seems to disappear one kilometre at a time.

I approached the riverbank for the last time, knowing I didn't have to do it again and after this bit was done it was just a case of pushing to the end. I knew that each step forward was a testament to my endurance, as I embraced the raw and untamed energy that coursed through the fields with every gust.

I was proud of myself that despite the anxiety I experienced in the first part of the marathon, I kept running, and I ran the whole way without stopping. I didn't hit the wall. This time I was prepared: taking gels at regular intervals and drinking enough helped me push through. I also took two salt tablets during the race. I expected to see more people out and about during this marathon but, perhaps because of the strong winds, people opted to walk in the village instead of next to the open fields. I did see two ladies I see during most of my runs, and because of that in a way it felt like any other Sunday long run.

When I had only 700 metres left to go, I called Paul and asked him to go home and wait for me there. I ran those last 700 metres with pride, but I didn't have the mental strength to push myself any harder. I was afraid that if I made a mistake, I wouldn't be able to finish. Even though I had plenty of energy left in the tank, I was afraid to give it everything I had. When my watch finally showed 26.2 miles, I abruptly stopped running, even though I was still 100 metres away from home. I collapsed on the ground, tears streaming down my face, but I was overjoyed to be part of the 1% of the world's population who have successfully completed a marathon.

When I finally arrived home, my husband and son greeted me with cheers and congratulations. Although I hadn't hit the original time goal I secretly set myself, I had achieved something truly amazing. I had finished a marathon in under 5 hours: in 4 hours and 47 minutes.

Running a marathon is not only an athletic achievement but also a mental achievement that requires a strong state of mind. I proved this to myself by completing my first marathon solo in a virtual race on a windy day. Despite my busy schedule, I trained thrice weekly for five months to prepare for the race. During this time, I transitioned from being a meat eater to a vegetarian and eventually adopted a wholly plant-based diet. Although I experienced self-doubt, I maintained my belief in myself and reminded myself that even if I wasn't happy with my pace or effort, I was still doing more than the majority of people who were simply sitting on their couch watching TV.

I have done it. I have run a marathon.

Chapter 9:
Aftermath of the Marathon

The finish line is just the beginning of a whole new race – the race to recover, to refocus, to recharge, and to start all over again.

Unknown

As soon as I finished my marathon, I wanted to run another one, only better. I really wanted to, but my training load heavily decreased for various reasons.

Although I felt ready to run after just one day of rest, I decided to wait three full days before attempting to run again. On the fourth day, I went for a 5k run but started feeling slight discomfort in my left hip after running just over 3k. I walked for about 300–400 metres before picking up my pace again, feeling fine for the remainder of the distance.

Despite the initial high, emotionally I was feeling entirely down after completing my marathon, and it was difficult for me to express those feelings. The internet suggested that booking another race would help. I tried to follow the advice and find another marathon, but the options were limited due to the ongoing Covid-19 restrictions. The overachiever in me wasn't pleased with how my marathon went. I performed well, but deep down, I wasn't satisfied. I also didn't want to run another marathon solo. As a result, my confidence was shaken, and I was hesitant to tackle another marathon on my own.

The pride of my marathon triumph was tinged with a disappointment that lingered in me for a week after the event. On the one hand I had the urge to tell anyone and everyone, even strangers, about my achievement; on the other I still couldn't shake the feeling of being down. While Paul tried to console me by reminding me that I had done great, I struggled to overcome my disappointment. His words that my feat was no longer new news to others and that great news quickly became yesterday's news were a reminder that life moves on. However, I knew deep down that finishing a marathon was something to be proud of, regardless of external validation. Ultimately, I decided to focus on the journey I had taken to get to that point and the satisfaction of crossing the finish line.

I tried to pick myself up, and on the Saturday following my marathon we departed for a lovely seaside holiday in Norfolk. The weather wasn't great, but I was looking forward to some time off with my family. I was sure the seaside walks and runs would make me feel better.

During that holiday, I had the opportunity to run three times, and Norfolk runs taught me something new about myself, including how to be present and embrace the weather conditions, no matter what they were like. On one run, I learned how to handle running in the wind. On my third run of the week, I surprised myself by setting a personal best (PB) for 5k, even though the first section was on sand. I felt like I was flying. The wind was in my favour during that run, but on the way back, I faced wind and rain that slowed me down. Nevertheless, I felt happy and content, reassured that much of my difficulty during the marathon was due to the strong winds.

Upon returning home from the holiday, however, I found that I could not run at my desired pace and distance. My usual route, which I had previously enjoyed, now seemed repetitive and uninteresting. I also experienced stomach problems during some of my longer runs. On top of all this, I fell ill with a bug that Jacob had picked up from preschool, which further hindered my training. I felt exhausted and out of it. I think my body just needed some rest.

When I started to feel better, I started running again. That short running break did me good and I suddenly felt motivated again. I signed up for a 1,000-km challenge just a few days after the marathon, which required me to run just over 621 miles within a calendar year. I was able to use all the miles I had done since April and I was delighted to reach 1,000 km at the beginning of November, which was a significant achievement for me, particularly considering my previous non-existent level of physical activity. During those seven months, I ran more than I ever had in my entire life. That milestone showed me that I had transformed into a dedicated runner.

But still with no races to look forward to, I sought another challenge to motivate myself. I set my sights on completing the

'John o'Groats to Lands End Virtual Challenge'. This required me to run a total of 874 miles during the year – the distance between the bottom (Land's End) and the top (John o'Groats) of the UK – by the end of the year. Since I didn't even start running until the middle of April, I'd already lost the first few months of the year to complete this challenge, and I had less than two months to cover 252 miles.

The final months of that year turned out to be my highest mileage months, despite the various challenges life threw at me. At the beginning of December, Jacob's teacher contracted Covid-19, and the whole class had to self-isolate for fourteen days. This was a difficult time for me emotionally. I struggled to go back to lockdown vibes and maintain healthy eating habits, and I ended up having more wine than usual. Meanwhile, Paul was very busy at work due to his increased workload during Covid-19, which meant that my only option was to run any longer mileage during the weekends and the very early hours of the day during the week.

I started running in the dark, which was something I hadn't done before. For someone who is scared of darkness, our village looked eerie, with limited street lights, so I had to run back and forth on the main street, making a half-mile loop. It was boring, but I did it to get the necessary mileage. I was also experiencing various physical niggles, such as knee pain and pain under my foot. I put it down to my worn-out shoes, so, after 500 miles I retired my reliable first pair of Mizunos and replaced them with a new pair. I felt emotional, as these shoes had been through so much with me and were the ones I used for marathon training and to get my first PBs.

However, switching to a new pair of trainers proved to be a game changer. They felt like I was running on clouds, and I started to run faster. I could even run negative splits during my long runs, which I had never done before, and I set a new half marathon PB of 2 hours and 7 minutes (a PB that still remains to this date). In hindsight, I don't believe the new shoes helped me run faster. Instead, I think it was the many slow, lower heart rate miles that I completed during my Lands End to John o'Groats challenge. Those slow miles helped me build endurance and strength, allowing me to run faster and longer distances without getting tired quickly.

I focused on my mileage during the challenge without worrying about my pace. I had some beautiful long runs where I could let my mind wander and enjoy the scenery. During those runs, I wrote part of this book in my head and began to believe that anything was possible and that good things would come to me. I was grateful for the opportunity to participate in the challenge, as it helped me rekindle my passion for running that had become extinguished in my post-marathon low; it reminded me of the many positive things it brought to my life.

I completed the John o'Groats to Lands End challenge just a few days before the end of 2020, and reaching that target was an incredible feeling. It was a reminder that with dedication and perseverance, I could overcome any obstacle. It was a way for me to end the year on a positive note, start the new year with a renewed sense of motivation and purpose, and continue with a newfound joy of running.

PART II:
A YEAR OF SETBACKS

Chapter 10:
When Your Body Doesn't Work with You

Tough Times Never Last, But Tough People Do!

ROBERT SCHULLER

It was a cold and rainy Sunday morning in January, and it was time for my weekly long run. Whatever the weather, I always look forward to my runs, especially on Sunday mornings. However, that day felt different. I stared out the window several times, looking at the dark, dreary rain. As I hesitated to go, I decided to do an hour on the indoor bike before starting my run.

Like a true athlete, I felt empowered as I pushed through my bike session. After finishing, I changed into my running gear and headed out the door. Unfortunately, my excitement was short-lived as I quickly realised that the rain had turned to snow and ice, which made running impossible. Disappointed, I returned home, changed into dry clothes, and decided to do another hour on the bike instead. Despite the second bike session being more challenging than the first, I was proud of myself for still managing to complete a long cardio session regardless of the unexpected weather.

Eager to hit the pavement for a run, I looked forward to my next session on Tuesday. The weather, yet again, had other plans. Although I'd rather run, having cycled during my last session, I knew I needed to maintain my fitness routine, so I braced myself for another indoor ride. When it was time for my next session on Thursday, the conditions were still icy, so I had no choice but to cycle again. I had been running for nine months, but I still had doubts about my ability to run. I don't know why I was thinking that all those long runs that I had completed were just a blip. At that moment, I started to seriously question if I was capable of running at all. Silly, right? I could easily cycle 20 miles, but I had doubts about my ability to run any distance, however short. It's interesting how self-doubt can be so persistent.

During that third bike session, I pushed myself to the limit. As I got off the bike I felt a nagging pain under my foot. This was not an unfamiliar feeling, as I had experienced the same nagging pain in December after some of my early morning runs. Back then, I thought it was because my trainers were wearing out, which is when I switched to the new pair. I also iced my foot after the runs and massaged it with a spiky ball. The pain always went away before my next run, and I considered the problem solved.

So when I felt this pain again, after three bike sessions, I didn't give it much thought and went about my day. A few days

CHAPTER 10: WHEN YOUR BODY DOESN'T WORK WITH YOU • 93

later, however, the pain had worsened. Despite trying all of my usual methods to ice, elevate, and rest to alleviate the pain, I saw no improvement. My old friend spiky ball only made things worse and as the days passed, the pain increased. Then the ball of my foot swelled up and turned red. I couldn't put my finger on what had caused this. The pain was so bad that I struggled to sleep, even with painkillers.

My running journey had started off great, and I felt unstoppable after completing the Lands End to John o'Groats challenge. I had been looking forward to what 2021 had in store for me, but my excitement turned out to be short-lived as I faced this injury, even though I'd incorporated strength training into my running routine from the beginning.

In hindsight, I shouldn't have gone so hard on the bike when I couldn't run due to the icy outdoor conditions. But since at this point we didn't have a treadmill at home, running indoors wasn't an option. It had been a few months since my last cycling session, and I'd charged ahead with too much enthusiasm. However, since I am a stubborn person and running is the one thing that keeps me going and helps me deal with everything else in my life, I thought that by maintaining my fitness with cycling, I would be able to resume running in no time. The pain under the ball of my foot had other plans for me. My strong desire to run again wasn't enough; I struggled with the fact that I couldn't. It was challenging to come to terms with an injury stopping me from doing what I loved.

I tried to steer to other activities. A year before I started running, I immersed myself in fluid art. Every opportunity

I had, I would play with my paints and experimented with techniques I had seen other artists using. When the lockdown started, I lost interest. Bright colours and the opportunity to create didn't seem to fill my cup any more. Being injured motivated me to pick up my art again, but with Jacob being home from preschool that month, I struggled to find uninterrupted stretches of time to do fluid art. So I explored other techniques that I could do alongside him and just painted. In the evenings I tried to read, but I just wasn't able to concentrate on a book for long enough. During times like these, I binge-watch box sets of medical dramas and crime shows. I struggle to concentrate on movies; series are just right. Somehow, it helps until I feel I can cope again.

But I missed running. I missed the alone time that running provided me and the sense of accomplishment. Instead of taking time to heal properly, I pushed through. After a few weeks, I managed the pain with the help of kinesiology tape and physio exercises, which I found on the internet. I slowly started running again, starting with walk/run intervals and gradually built up my endurance.

By mid-February I'd made progress with my running and started pushing myself to go for longer distances. Then without warning, we lost our beloved dog, Stanley. The house felt empty without him, and I struggled to explain his absence to Jacob. The book I bought to help explain what happens to animals when they die – *Megan's Journey* by Janet Peel – ended up making me even more emotional. It contained a beautiful story about a dog that had passed away, finding solace at the rainbow bridge with her late brother. In the narrative, both pups are sitting by the lake of love, looking back at their family, sending beautiful white feathers to remind them that they had arrived safely and were thinking about them. To this day, I can't read this book without tearing up. Jacob continues to collect white feathers, which bring us both great comfort.

I sensed myself slipping back into the unwelcome company of my old friend, depression. I knew that running wouldn't bring Stanley back, but I also knew a nice long run would help me to process his loss. So I decided I really wanted to run in his memory. Though I was now running a bit further my mileage was still low. Instead of being sensible and running a shorter distance, I went all out and ran 15 miles for him (a mile for each year he was with us). The sensible thing would have been to run 15k, but I thought that Stanley was a British dog, not Estonian, so I went all in and ran 15 miles. The run was emotionally significant as I reminisced about our time together and envisioned him running alongside me, even though in reality we never ran together, due to his age.

Stanley had been my companion when I first moved to England, providing me with constant company and unconditional love. I didn't realise how much I missed him until he was gone. In addition to the intense sadness I felt, I also experienced a sense of guilt and regret. I couldn't help but wonder if there was anything more I could have done to keep him with us longer. Maybe if we had caught his illness sooner, he would still be here with us. These thoughts weighed heavily on my heart, and I found myself struggling to come to terms with his passing.

Mentally, this run gave me peace. But physically, it was definitely too big a jump while I was recovering from my foot injury. I also felt some pressure and tightness in my knee during my run but carried on. By the time I'd finished the run, the pain was intense. I iced my knee and thought I would carry on as normal in a few days.

My subsequent runs started off well, but the pain was never far behind, always making an appearance. It was unpredictable and would surface unexpectedly during runs, causing me to cut my runs short or walk home. The pleasure of running slowly faded away as I constantly worried about when the pain would arise. All of this led to a sense of frustration. Strangely, dealing with the emotional and mental aspects of running injuries was more difficult than dealing with the physical pain. Running injuries can be dreadful, as they make you question everything. Running was my solitude, and it just didn't feel fair that I wasn't able to run. After trying everything I could to resolve the injury independently, I decided to book a visit to see a sports physiotherapist.

It wasn't my first visit to a sports physio. From my very first lockdown runs, I had a recurring knee niggle, but as it always eased when I warmed up, I never had to stop running. Paul thought that I would never book a session myself for just a niggle, so he gifted me a session after my marathon. During the session, she confirmed my runner's knee diagnosis and gave me some exercises, which I started a few days after my marathon. To be fair, these exercises helped, and I never experienced that type of knee pain again.

This time, I entered her office full of hope. She was sitting at her computer when I entered, and as she got up to greet me, I couldn't help but notice her athletic runner's body. I thought she was so lucky to know exactly what to do for any running problem she might face – I even felt a slight twinge of jealousy.

'How can I help?' she asked in a friendly voice.

'I think it's my IT band,' I answered. I had done my research back home, and I was pretty sure that's what was wrong. The internet said it could take up to six weeks to recover, so I was hoping she knew something I didn't. I just wasn't ready to accept it and was looking for her to perform some sort of miracle that would get me back to running like normal without taking time off.

She asked where exactly the pain is and told me to lay on her table. 'Yep, it's your IT band. It is really tight here,' she said, massaging the side of my thigh while I winced with pain. When she was finished, she applied bright pink kinesiology tape.

'Can I run?' I asked anxiously.

'Well, you shouldn't run when you feel pain,' she answered.

Still trying to negotiate, I carried on, 'But it never hurts at the beginning of the run: it starts to hurt after a certain mileage.'

She said, 'You should always stop before it starts hurting.' Then added, 'You could always cross-train.' She then promised to email across my exercises and booked me in for another session in a few weeks' time. I followed the prescribed plan to the letter but still didn't see improvements.

All of it had the opposite effect. I had a good routine before becoming injured. When I saw the physio the first time, I added exercises for runner's knee to my existing practice. Then when I got my foot injury, yet another set of exercises was added to my routine. Before seeing her for my IT band pain, I'd added exercises that I found from my own research. Now I had another set to add. It was a lot. I used to do strength training and physio exercises three times a week. I had to do these new exercises daily. I was struggling to fit it all in, and I was just getting bored. I just wanted to run like I used to! I started to get fed up and dislike any kind of strength training and physio.

During my period of injury, I never fully stopped running, which was my downfall, really. I probably would have recovered a lot better if I had given my body what it needed the most – rest. Instead, I pushed it until it hurt and then was upset that it hurt. I just couldn't accept that all those good emotions I got from running during 2020 had to be put on pause.

Running can elicit a plethora of positive emotions, but I have come to realise that during times of injury, it can also bring about many negatives. When I was actively running, any negative emotions seemed to fade away during my runs, and I was left with a heightened sense of positivity. However, being injured is not easy. Sometimes, I found myself in a bad mood for no apparent reason, feeling really low. While it wasn't directly because of my inability to run like I used to, not being able to engage in the activity that brought me joy certainly didn't help.

As I was writing this book, I found myself wondering whether 'runner's low' was a term I had just made up or whether others experienced it as well. A quick Google search confirmed that many runners do indeed experience it, and I can certainly relate many of my running experiences during the first part of 2021 to runner's low. I often experienced runner's low when I had to stop running due to pain. Suddenly, what was once a joyful experience became a source of worry. I found myself wondering how far I would be able to go before the pain set in, and how I would manage to get my exercise in if the pain became too much to bear. Those moments were incredibly frustrating and made running feel like more of a chore than a source of enjoyment.

The weight of it all made me feel incredibly down. The feeling of heaviness in my chest due to my ongoing injury frustrations became constant. I have a depressive nature that never entirely goes away; running just helps to manage it. I recognised its evil head lurking in the shadows. I desperately wanted to start feeling better and get back to doing what I love.

Depression is something I've grappled with since my teenage years. I never believed I was good enough, smart enough, pretty enough, or skinny enough. Just never enough. I seemed to be out of sync with the world around me. As my teenage years began, I attempted to stand out and be different, hoping it would make me feel unique enough to fit into the 'different enough' category. I adorned myself in outrageously colourful clothes, dyed my hair in shades of red and blue, and just wanted to fit in in my own way.

Over the years, I've learned to coexist with my unwelcome companion, experiencing both better and worse periods.

Whenever I'm unable to run due to injury or illness, I feel the onset of the unwelcome shadow of depression. Being injured has tested me countless times, as running is my usual remedy for stress and anxiety. Without it, I am forced to dig deep and find other ways to cope.

Chapter 11:
Running Is Cheaper Than Therapy

When I ran, some of the anxiety, depression, and mania dropped away. Running helped me focus, calmed me, gave me a sense of accomplishment, and brought joy. It allowed me to achieve small goals.

NITA SWEENEY

I had now been struggling with knee pain for a while, and I was constantly worried it would start during my run. Instead of the road where I usually ran, I opted to run on a soft surface, such as grass or a dirt road – mainly grass to lessen the impact on my knees. I really wanted to run longer this time, but I knew I probably wouldn't get past the 8k mark as that's where the pain typically started. I had been feeling down about myself and my running, but during this sunny spring run, despite my worries, I felt like I was on top of the world, at the top of my running game. It was the first short-sleeved run of the year, and the weather was lovely and sunny. It would have been a shame to miss it.

It was the end of March, a time that holds a special place in my heart. One of my favourite moments of the year, when nature undergoes a magical transformation. I delight in the sight of daffodils gracefully emerging along roadsides. The grass, now adorned in a vibrant hue, is becoming noticeably greener, and there's a general sense of lushness in the outdoors. It's a season that breathes life into the surroundings, bringing with it the promise of renewal and the awakening of nature's beauty.

Changing my running from road to off-road gave me a different perspective on my running. As soon as I reached the beck, I had to put my long-sleeved top back on since the wind was relatively strong, and I felt cold. I hadn't taken a drink with me as I feared that carrying a drink in my right hand might contribute to my left leg problems. In the past, I had tried holding the water bottle in each hand, but it always ended up in my right hand. Carrying it in my left hand just felt oddly wrong. I didn't use my hydration vest for shorter runs; it was easier to fill up the bottle.

I simply kept running, enjoying the beautiful scenery around me. To my right was the fast-flowing beck and to my left were fields as far as the eye could see. As I approached a bench on the other side of the beck in front of some woods, I wondered who might use it. There didn't seem to be an obvious way to get to the other side, and most dog walkers stuck to the same side of the beck that I was on. I promised myself that once I felt confident that I could run long enough without pain, I would run to the other side to find out. I didn't see anyone else that day. When the beck joined the river, I knew I should turn back, but I couldn't resist the urge to keep running.

As I ran across Cadney Bridge, I noticed something resembling a running vest on the railings. As I got closer, I saw the words 'Caistor Running Club' printed on it. The vest served as a poignant memorial to a fellow runner who had tragically taken his own life in the river below the month before. Although I had never met him, I couldn't help but feel a deep sense of sadness and wonder about what had led him to make such a devastating decision.

As I continued to run, my thoughts turned to my own struggles with depression, a battle I've been fighting for as long as I can remember. I've had dark moments where I've felt like giving up on life. However, I've been lucky to have people in my life who were able to support me and make sure I was okay. But depression is an insidious disease, and it never really goes away. I've learned to live with and manage it, but it's always there in the background, waiting to rear its ugly head again. It's a disease that too many people suffer from, often hidden behind a facade of smiles and laughter. It's a chilling thought that we can never really know what's going on inside someone else.

Like Nita Sweeney, I find comfort from depression by running.[2] Running is cheaper than therapy, and it works better for some than others. Since I started running, I have noticed that my depressive episodes are more manageable. Many of my issues can be resolved with the long run. It may sound like a cliché, but it really works for me. I believe any kind of exercise helps with depression, whether it's a long walk, yoga session, cardio workout, or running. Exercise has genuinely helped me.

Back in January 2021, while struggling with my foot injury, I was hit by a major emotional blow when my father passed away from Covid-19.

My relationship with my father was never an easy one. We never shared a close bond, and from my childhood, I have few memories of him. I recall him spending most of his time in his 'man cave' in the garage. I couldn't say what he was doing there, he never shared that with us. He felt like a stranger living in our home alongside me, my sister, my mum, and my grandma.

After my parents' divorce, he moved to a small flat outside of town. He didn't visit often, and when he did, it always felt awkward, leaving me unsure about how to feel toward him. Later on in life, he made some attempts to build a relationship, but it was apparent that his motives were primarily selfish, driven by a desire to ensure that I understood my obligation to care for him in his old age.

His passing left me with a mix of confusing emotions. At a time when I needed mental clarity the most, running was not an option, and the loss of my father affected me more deeply than I expected. We had been estranged for years, and I still harboured many negative feelings towards him. When my sister called to tell me our father had tested positive for Covid-19, I didn't give it much thought and took a pragmatic approach. A few days later, on his seventy-eighth birthday, he was hospitalised. His condition worsened from there, and he passed away two weeks later. During his hospitalisation, I talked with my sister a lot, and in a way, his illness brought us closer together.

CHAPTER 11: RUNNING IS CHEAPER THAN THERAPY

After his passing, I didn't know how to process my thoughts and feelings about him. I was always taught that you shouldn't speak ill of the dead, but I had a lot of unresolved feelings about him and our relationship. When people offered their condolences, I felt like a fraud because I didn't feel like I had the right to grieve due to our non-existent relationship in the years leading up to his death.

With my injury leaving me incapable of running, I felt I didn't have access to the form of therapy that I had come to know so well, which could usually help me untangle my thoughts. My husband was amazing! Even though our son couldn't attend preschool that month, he made time from his busy work schedule to take further care of him, which allowed me to go out for the walk/runs that my injury allowed and get some much-needed outdoor time. I wanted to do a run in my father's memory, but at that time I couldn't even run 7.8k. Instead, a year later, I completed a run in his memory, running 7.8 miles in total. It was a quiet and private run. One that I ran just for me and my dad. It felt liberating to finally do what I do best: finding comfort in running.

When our dog Stanley passed away, which I mentioned in the previous chapter, I was overwhelmed with sadness. The loss of my father in my mind followed by losing Stanley was a painful reminder of the impermanence of life and the importance of cherishing every moment we have with our loved ones.

There are days when I lack the motivation to run, particularly during my low-mood periods. I find that I really want to run, but my pessimistic thoughts hold me back. If I skip the run, I find myself beating myself up. Fortunately, there are things that I can do that work. When I feel that I can't run, I know I can cycle. I am lucky to have the option to escape to our garden shed, spend some time on my trusty exercise bike, and watch something on my tablet that distracts me from my racing negative thoughts.

Running in the mornings helps me get started and sets a positive tone for the day. By the end of the day, I often feel drained and the thought of running seems unappealing. If I already feel down and haven't managed to exercise in the morning, it's quite likely that my run won't happen. Although I know that a run would benefit me, the idea of relaxing on the couch with snacks or getting an early night feels more enticing. Yet if I wake up the following day, lace up my shoes and head out for a run, suddenly the world feels like a better place again. I know that if I stick to my running routine, there will be more good days, and I am just happy to be running whether the sun shines or the rain pours.

Running for me is not just about the physical aspect, but also the mental and emotional benefits it provides. It's my time to meditate, get relief from stress, dream, and sadly grieve. It's a form of therapy for me, a way to cope with life's challenges and to find peace in difficult times. Running is cheaper than therapy, and it's something that I will continue to turn to whenever I need it. Being denied running only highlighted more clearly how much it helps me.

Chapter 12:
Rebound

Fall down seven times, stand up eight.

Japanese proverb

As my birthday in July approached, I realised with a heavy heart that I had been on and off injured for nearly six long months and was struggling to stay positive. I had managed to build my runs back up to 10k, but I couldn't run any further without crippling pain in my knee. Negative thoughts began to creep in, and I blamed myself for not doing enough to speed up my recovery.

I noticed that my thoughts were getting more and more overwhelming. I craved to follow my training plans, but my injury had made it impossible. I used to find such joy in setting distance goals during my long runs, and the sense of satisfaction I felt when I achieved them was indescribable. Now, that option just wasn't available, and I hadn't been able to do it since January.

After being plagued by injuries for six months, I reached a breaking point. I had been asking myself, *Why me?* I was eating well, doing various exercises, and generally being sensible, so I couldn't understand why my knee injury wasn't healing and had no idea what I could do differently. It all left me feeling down and distraught. All I wanted was to run again. Since I was already doing physically as much as possible to overcome my injury, I focused on the mental aspect and did everything I could to improve my mental strength. That's when I stumbled upon the book *Rebound: Train Your Mind to Bounce Back Stronger from Sports Injuries* by Carrie Jackson Cheadle and Cindy Kuzma.

I started following the mental exercises outlined in the book and was amazed at its positive impact on my recovery. *Rebound* gave me a different perspective on my injuries, and instead of feeling sad about what I couldn't do and comparing my accomplishments to those from the past, I began to look at things in a new way and started fresh. I started to celebrate my achievements from that moment forward. Whenever I could complete a 5k run without experiencing any pain, I treated it as a triumph. I celebrated it regardless of whether it was slower than my previous runs or shorter than my usual distance. Whilst working through the book, I took a week off from running altogether to re-evaluate my approach to physical activity. I upped my cycling and permitted myself to enjoy it. That following week I cycled 91 miles, including my longest ride on my indoor bike: 39 miles for my thirty-ninth birthday. (I had hoped to run 39 miles for my thirty-ninth birthday, but as my injury did not subside I realised it was just a dream. Instead of forgetting this dream, I kept my dream alive by planning to run 40 miles for my fortieth birthday the next summer.)

It took much effort to address the mental aspect of my injuries, but I believe it played a crucial role in my recovery. I took the advice of the book and worked on managing my emotions. I completed most of the exercises it provided, including a SWOT analysis of my injury, and an injury intake form. I even wrote a 'get well' card for myself. Through these exercises, I shifted my mindset from feeling like a victim and trying to control everything to a more empowered and positive outlook. I had been plagued by self-doubt, wondering how I would ever be able to run another marathon when I was struggling even to run 6 miles. A change of thinking was pushing those thoughts aside, and as my mental outlook shifted, my physical body seemed to follow suit.

But while my knee was now improving, I continued to experience pain under the ball of my foot after runs. I had done what I could on my own to resolve it, with not much difference, so I decided to see a podiatrist; that meeting turned out to be a game changer. I had never seen a podiatrist before, and I really didn't know what to expect. I took my trainers with me to show what I ran in. As I waited, my glasses kept steaming up. I still hadn't got used to wearing a mask with my glasses, but I didn't have a choice; it was a requirement. As per the request when I booked the appointment I was wearing shorts.

The podiatrist asked me to sit on the sofa and carefully examined my feet. Suddenly, she asked, 'Could you show me your hands?' As I reached my hands out, she asked me to push my thumb back to touch my forearm. It seemed like an odd request, but I did it with no issues. After examining my hands, she examined my feet again and said, 'I think you have hypermobility.' I had never heard of it. She explained, 'It's a fairly common condition and it's not really an illness. It just means your joints are more flexible than they should be. I have it too.'

I could have asked so many questions, but my mind went blank and I brushed it off as something common that I just have.

'I'm going to make you some insoles for your trainers,' she said, before leaving to make them. As I was sitting there barefoot and waiting for her return, I was feeling hopeful. At least I knew what was wrong with me.

As she returned, she asked, 'What brand are your trainers?' I was wearing my Mizuno Wave Rider Osakas for the appointment. At first sight, there is nothing special about those trainers, but one trainer has a different colour scheme than the other. Although they don't scream colour, they are just colourful enough, and everyone who sees them thinks I am wearing trainers from different pairs. I felt smug about my trainer choice; I loved that particular pair of trainers that brought me many compliments over the years. Those trainers were such fun!

She sent me home with a pair of orthotics, which didn't look particularly special – just a pair of insoles without much padding. The orthotics provided a great deal of relief initially. Although I used them a lot during the next months, I don't use them any more. I have since opted for a softer, over-the-counter pair of Enertor insoles instead.

After my podiatrist diagnosed me with hypermobility, I went home and researched it to learn more about the condition. Suddenly, everything started to make sense. I had been frustrated with my long-term injury, and how, despite following all the right steps, I wasn't recovering as quickly as I had hoped. But now, having a reason for my slow recovery progress was a relief. Understanding my body's limitations with hypermobility helped me adjust my expectations and approach my recovery differently. Within a few weeks, I found that I was enjoying cycling more and more, and I was even able to run again like I used to. Although I experienced some discomfort from my orthotics, I was elated that I could run.

I now accept that I may always be prone to injury, but I am determined to build my training around it. Injuries don't define who I am as a runner. Instead, they have made me stronger and more resilient. Every time I've faced an injury, I've had to dig deep and find the mental strength to push through the setbacks and return stronger. The road to recovery may not be easy, but it has taught me the value of perseverance, determination, and self-care. I have learned that caring for my body and mind is just as important as training hard; that setbacks are not the end but a necessary part of growth and improvement. Becoming more mindful of my body and how it responds to different types of training means I have adjusted my approach accordingly to prevent future injuries.

Injuries have also given me a new perspective on what it means to be a runner. Instead of solely focusing on speed and distance, I have come to appreciate the process, the small victories along the way, and the mental strength it takes to overcome adversity. I am grateful for the lessons I have learned through my injuries and how they have made me a better, more resilient runner. Yes, injuries may have been a part of my running journey, but they don't define me. Instead, they have made me stronger and more determined to reach my goals.

Chapter 13:
Back in the Game

*If it is important to you, you will find a way.
If not, you'll find an excuse.*

RYAN BLAIR

After my first marathon I knew I wanted to run another one. Hoping to make the experience easier, I aimed to do an in-person race for my second marathon. I looked into several local marathons, but quite a few still weren't taking place. Since I couldn't find anything suitable, I decided to leave it, hoping that I would find the right marathon when the time was right.

In March, despite still recovering from injury, I still really wanted to run another marathon. I reasoned that signing up for one would provide me with something to look forward to and would make my injury recovery easier. I thought that by the time the serious training started, I would be fully recovered. While contemplating the prospect of another virtual race, an advertisement for the Virtual London Marathon seized my attention. Its slightly earlier timing meant my training time was more limited than I would have liked, but I couldn't shake the idea.

I shared my thought process with Paul. Sensing my excitement, he said, 'You will regret it if you don't do it. Maybe it will be the last virtual marathon they will do.'

I still wasn't entirely sold, thinking that an in-person race would be better – I tend to overthink and be rather cautious. Over the next few days, I envisioned having the London Marathon medal and T-shirt and I entered.

I signed up in faith that the ambitious marathon goal would serve as a powerful mental motivator during my recovery from injury. However, as reality unfolded, it became apparent that instead of providing the mental support I had hoped for, the marathon commitment added an unexpected layer of pressure.

Despite my strong desire to engage in rigorous training, my ambitions were thwarted by the persistent pain in my knee, courtesy of iliotibial band syndrome, which had been confirmed by the physio. I longed to follow my marathon training plans, to push my limits and prepare for the upcoming challenges. The nagging discomfort in my knee proved unyielding, casting a shadow over my enthusiasm. I had not yet had my revelatory appointment with the podiatrist, nor had I done the work on my resilience and mindset, so at this point I felt utterly in the dark about why my injury wasn't healing.

It was disheartening to feel the weight of my own physical limitations hindering my desire for training. Every attempt to lace up my running shoes and do what my training plan said was met with a reminder of the lingering pain. The frustration of wanting to push myself but being held back by the unrelenting discomfort left me dispirited. In those moments, I couldn't help but feel disappointed and I longed for the invigorating sensation of a fulfilling workout.

The marathon was getting closer, but my injury still persisted. 'I should be recovered by now!' I said to anyone who asked about my injury. My marathon goal was always in the back of my mind and it frustrated me that I had to stop and start my training and that I wasn't able to follow my training plan. I had to replace many of my runs with cycling sessions and there were many times when I doubted if I could ever run a full marathon. Talk about keeping all your eggs in one basket: I didn't have any other upcoming races scheduled that year, so I saw the marathon as an opportunity to challenge myself and run that one race that counts.

After seeing the podiatrist, however, things started to brighten up. Despite still experiencing knee pain, things changed around quickly. My perseverance paid off and eventually I was able to pick up and follow my training plan for the time I had left. But with only two months left until the marathon, time was running out to prepare for the race fully.

Initially, I had intended to follow a more rigorous marathon training plan from MarathonPal.com. After a frank assessment of my current fitness level, I realised that it wasn't feasible for me this time. Instead, I opted to revisit the novice programme that had helped me achieve success for my first marathon. It gave me the guidance and structure my training needed. As someone who thrives on visual progress, I printed out the training plan and enjoyed checking off the completed sessions. The first part of my training plan looked bare, but instead of concentrating on what I wasn't able to do, I focused on what I *was* able. I missed quite a few of my running sessions, but once I added my cycling to the plan it didn't look that bad. It was reassuring to see that my training had not been entirely derailed, and I remained optimistic about my marathon prospects.

During that period, I often reflected on my first marathon training experiences and felt discouraged by the prospect of falling short. I tried to push these thoughts aside and focus on the progress I had made this year. Although I had not logged as many running miles as the first time, I had incorporated a significant amount of cross-training into my routine and I was generally feeling fit.

As the marathon date drew closer, I realised that I needed to carefully consider my fuelling strategy during the race. Looking back at my notes from my first marathon, I recall using gels every 45 minutes, consuming a banana before starting the race, and taking one salt tablet before and two during the race. It was a successful approach at the time. When I trained for my first marathon I mostly ran in the early mornings, straight from bed, or in the evenings, a few hours after having my evening meal. However, that year I had been running more during my son's school hours, which meant running after breakfast. While running on an empty stomach had worked well for me the previous year, I had been struggling with it a bit more while training for the Virtual London Marathon. Simply eating a banana before my run no longer seemed to be sufficient.

And so, I remained undecided on how I would fuel during the race that year. I hadn't had much opportunity to practise on my longer runs, and I had used fewer gels and more natural food during my training runs. While I had hoped to steer clear of gels altogether, they were convenient and worked well for me. On the other hand, I wondered if it was wise to try something new when I already had a proven formula that had worked in the past.

I was really hoping to achieve a good time for my second marathon, but there were a few factors that would affect my performance. Weather and anxiety played a significant role in my first marathon. This year, the weather looked to be slightly better, although it was still expected to be windy. I was hesitant to change my route due to the wind, as I'd already envisioned the route I wanted to take.

As I reviewed my training data, I noticed that my pace had slowed somewhat compared to my previous performances at the end of 2020, but I was still showing an improvement over my pace compared to my first marathon training in the middle part of 2020. Despite this, I remained determined to achieve my goal of completing a marathon in under 4 hours and 30 minutes. To accomplish this, I reminded myself to give my maximum effort and believe in my ability to perform at my current level of training. I recognised that I had much work to do in the remaining two months leading up to the marathon and that it was critical for me to prioritise injury prevention as part of my training plan.

My newfound love for cycling definitely played a significant role in getting me to where I was with my training. The good weather didn't hurt, either. I gradually started incorporating more running into my routine – starting with shorter runs – and by mid-August, I was running three times a week, slowly building up my distance and speed. I was still cautious, not wanting to push too hard and risk re-injuring myself, but with each successful run, my confidence grew.

As I got closer to the virtual marathon date, I started to feel a mix of excitement and nervousness. I wasn't sure if I was fully prepared, but I was determined to give it my all.

Chapter 14:
Always a Lone Runner?

In the midst of difficulty lies opportunity.

ALBERT EINSTEIN

As I emerged from the bushes, I wondered, *Why am I even here in the first place?* It had started well: an advanced hills coaching session with the running club I was considering joining.

After a lengthy period of struggling with injuries that prevented me from pushing myself and improving, I found that I had lost much of the joy I used to feel when running. To keep myself motivated and feeling positive, I had to set different kinds of goals that would allow me to continue running and feeling good about my progress. As a result, just before my Virtual London Marathon in September 2021, I decided to join a local running club. I felt I just needed to change up my running.

Before joining the running club it had been years since I'd last run with someone else. Running alone had become my comfort zone ever since I started running during the first lockdown, and it was all I had ever known. Many moons ago, I occasionally ran with other people and completed a few short races, but I never really enjoyed it. I always went out too fast and tried to run other people's run, rather than my own. Even when I was running just with one other person, I didn't fully own that run; I was trying to keep up with them.

I was on time for my first session, and after introductions, we headed out for a gentle warm-up to the hills. After running 18 miles the weekend before, I entered the session confidently. 'Gentle' the coach had said. There were only two women in the group: me and one other lovely lady. The rest of the ten or so runners were men. I thought that at least I wasn't alone. But my relief was short-lived as it turned out the other lady was a speedy runner. I felt out of breath just over half a mile in.

I shouldn't have had water with dinner, I thought as I felt the familiar sensation of leaking. I apologised and headed to the bushes to check the damage, thoroughly embarrassed. She wanted to wait for me, but I encouraged her to carry on. When I got back to the road, everyone had gone. I just wanted to go home. I was new to the club but felt I would let everyone down if I disappeared. I didn't even have anyone's phone number to let them know. My only option was to accept my embarrassment and carry on with the session, hoping no one would notice my wet shorts. It was an unfamiliar route to me, and I didn't have my glasses with me (I am short-sighted and usually wear glasses for driving, but not running). Nevertheless, I decided to try to find my way.

I went in the direction I thought they had gone, which turned out to be wrong. I came back a bit and saw someone waving. Someone had been left behind to wait for me. I was glad I hadn't gone home! I apologised for wasting his time and said that I just needed to visit the bushes. It wasn't really a lie, but I couldn't really say what was actually wrong. He tried to make me feel better by saying that it's common to need the toilet during the runs. *Phew! He didn't notice my wet shorts*, I thought and breathed a sense of relief. We chatted about running as we continued to the hill.

It was a beast of a hill – muddy and steep, unlike anything I had ever encountered before. I was used to running in flat Lincolnshire, where what I considered to be hills weren't really hills at all. I was mostly running straight from my doorstep to make the most of the time available for me, on a fairly flat route. As I started running up and down the hill, I felt terrible. I struggled to keep up with the group, feeling out of my comfort zone and unsure if I belonged. I felt like I wasn't a proper runner. I tried to make the most of the downhills as much as I could and push up the hill, but unfortunately, it just wasn't my day. Then I saw Mike and Hannah (whom I knew from the running club) at the halfway point of the hill. They had just finished their own running session and had come to support the club runners. But instead of feeling encouraged, I felt like I needed to do a better job to deserve their support.

And to make things worse, my knee started to hurt, and I found myself limping more than running. At first, it was just a tightness in my hamstring that I had felt during my last few runs and so I brushed it off as nothing. But soon enough, the familiar crippling pain was back in my knee. *Not again!* I thought, as my run for that day finished. I limped up to the hill where my things were and then back down again with everyone else. I felt pathetic, a failure, holding everyone back, running less than everybody else and getting injured in the process. I just felt like I didn't belong with those seasoned runners.

I was relieved when the session was over, and I could get to my little car and drive away. I just wanted to cry. It was my worst run ever. I wasn't sure if I would ever run with another person again, yet alone the running group. Thankfully, after icing and rest, my knee pain disappeared, and four days later, I laced up and was running again on my own.

After my disappointing run, I considered quitting the running club altogether. However, I realised I shouldn't let one bad experience stop me from enjoying something I love. So I decided to give it another chance and attend another running club session. I was met with a group of friendly and supportive runners who welcomed me back with open arms. I swallowed my pride and overcame my initial feelings of embarrassment, realising that everyone has bad days and it's important to push past them.

I discovered that even if I run with other people, it's still my run. With more group running experience under my belt, I learned the importance of owning my runs. So now, whenever I run, I remind myself that I am in control and say to myself, *Merili, you own this run.* This simple sentence has tremendously improved my runs. I should have incorporated this mindset into that first group run, instead of letting imposter syndrome get the best of me.

These days, I still prefer to run alone at my own comfortable pace, but occasionally I run with a group of runners, where I can team up with any runner whose pace matches mine, and I can even feel great! Joining a running club brought a breath of fresh air into my life. I still worry about incontinence when I run with other people, but most of the time, the enjoyment of running with company beats it. Since then, I've had more fun runs with members of the club and have made some new friends. It's been a great reminder that so many lovely people in the running community share a passion for running and support each other through both the highs and lows. Running with such wonderful members from a running club even made me feel more like a real runner!

I had made the decision to broaden my knowledge of running, so I reached out to the friendly runners at the club. With their assistance, I successfully completed the England Athletics LiRF (Leadership in Running Fitness) and CiRF (Coach in Running Fitness) qualifications. My primary objective in learning more about running was to improve my own running abilities and avoid injuries in the future. A secondary benefit was knowing I'd be able to inspire and support others in accomplishing their running goals.

While I may not be a regular attendee at running club sessions, primarily due to family commitments and childcare responsibilities, being part of this welcoming club holds immense significance for me. I proudly wear my club vest and hoodie every time I participate in a race. The sense of belonging and camaraderie within the club resonates deeply with me, fostering a strong connection to the running community, and I always look forward to the times when I can fully immerse myself in the solidarity and shared passion for running that the sessions provide.

Chapter 15:
Virtual London Marathon

Pain is temporary, pride is forever.

Unknown

During the last 6 miles of my second marathon, I repeated the phrase 'pain is temporary, pride is forever' to myself as that all too familiar foot pain emerged. The pain was likely caused by the rubbing of my orthotics and my pre-existing injury in that area.

But before I got to race, I had to survive another tapering period. Tapering for my second marathon was a very different experience from the first. I started my taper earlier this time, running my 20-mile and final half marathon runs slightly ahead of schedule. Then, with only thirteen days until the marathon, I sat there with an ice pack on my knee. It felt slightly off during my cycling session the day before, but I ignored it as the pain wasn't too bad.

After learning about my hypermobility, I accepted that I needed to be mindful of how my body feels and be prepared to incorporate cross-training if required and plan time for strength training. The first half of the training cycle was marred with overcoming my knee pain, but during the second part of my marathon training cycle things worked well. So when I experienced niggles during the taper period, I was reluctant to accept it.

The taper for this marathon was another rollercoaster of emotions. I managed to run just twice during the two weeks leading up to the marathon due to having different pains and niggles. I replaced any missed runs with indoor cycling, but it wasn't the same as running. A few days before the marathon, I felt like a joke, icing three different areas on my leg and foot. To make matters worse, I was now suffering knee pain from activities as simple as walking the dog or just walking around the house. This made me think that my pains weren't real and were just caused by taper anxiety.

My time goal for this marathon was under 4 hours and 30 minutes, although I was uncertain if that was achievable. My training hadn't gone as planned, but I'd done my best to prepare: with some adjustments to the training plan I'd managed to get a decent amount of running in over the past two months and my recent half marathon results showed some promise. Ultimately, however, the outcome would depend on how the race day went. One thing was for sure: I didn't want to be slower than last year!

The weekend I was supposed to be doing my 20-mile run I was away from home, so I swapped the order of my 18-mile and 20-mile runs so that I did the 20-mile one followed by the 18-mile one. The 20-mile run went according to plan, but the day of my 18-mile run was a scorching day. I ran during the daytime and tried to find shade, but the heat got the better of me, and I had to stop at 15 miles. While I couldn't complete my 18-mile run due to the heat, I felt that running in hot conditions was still beneficial for my training. When you run in the heat, your body has to work harder to maintain its core temperature, which can improve your cardiovascular fitness and boost your endurance.

After being unable to complete the distance during my last long run, I had one more 13-mile run to complete, which turned out to be my best preparation for the marathon. I had planned to run it at a fast pace, but I went out too quickly at the beginning. Mid-run, I experienced a range of emotions and felt like giving up, as I found the pace challenging. However, I managed to slow down my pace and push through the tough moments. Later in the run, I managed to pick up the pace and ran some miles faster.

In the end, I was surprised to see it was my second-fastest half marathon time. This run gave me a lot of confidence for the upcoming marathon, knowing I could persevere through the tough moments and keep going. It reminded me of the importance of pacing and how mental strength is just as crucial as physical strength in long-distance running.

Despite experiencing some pains and niggles during my taper, I found myself more relaxed about things. It's common for old injuries and niggles to resurface during the taper period. All I could do was my best, and focus on what I could control. The anxiety I felt was normal before a big event, but it was different from the first time I ran a marathon. The first time, I was unsure if I could complete the distance, avoid hitting the wall, and run solo. This time I knew that I had the distance in me. In addition to my dodgy knee, foot pain, and possible shin splints, I'd had a runny nose for a week. My original plan included doing some fast interval sessions to improve my speed; none of it happened, as my body was not cooperating. While none of this was ideal, I had faith that everything would work out in the end. At times, it felt like my body had given up on me, and I was worried that I wouldn't be able to perform at my best during the marathon. However, I reminded myself that injuries and setbacks are a part of training and that it's essential to listen to my body and take care of it. The injury I experienced throughout the spring gave me a different perspective and, in a way, was a great teacher.

As the marathon approached, I was preoccupied with race-day clothing and checking the weather forecast. When I learned that strong winds were forecast for race day, I felt defeated and anxious. My first marathon had been run in similar conditions and I knew from my past running data that it would impact my performance. Although I couldn't control the weather, I still couldn't help but worry about how it would affect my race. I questioned whether running in windy conditions would be worse than running in hot weather. However, I focused on how the weather was beyond my control and it was still over a week until race day; the forecast could change many times between now and then.

Instead of setbacks, I concentrated on what I could control. I meditated and visualised myself running strong, feeling good, and achieving my goal of finishing the race in under 4 hours and 30 minutes. Instead of dwelling on the negative aspects of my training, I fixated on the positive. I focused on my progress and the hard work I had put in to get to this point. I celebrated the good days and stayed optimistic, even when things didn't go as planned. This shift in focus made me feel more empowered and in control of my training and mindset. It helped me approach the marathon with confidence and determination, knowing that I had done everything possible to prepare myself for success.

As marathon day approached, I prioritised rest and taking care of my body. I iced my knee and foot and made sure I stayed hydrated. I also ensured I ate well and got enough sleep in the days leading up to the race. My anxiety started to wear off a few days before the race, and I felt ready.

Just like with my first marathon, I wanted to start and finish my race at home. I diligently monitored the weather forecast, which had initially predicted those terrible conditions for the marathon, with strong winds and rain. However, as the marathon day drew nearer, the weather forecast started to improve. Until the weather forecast changed, I had even contemplated running the whole marathon in a 1.3k-loop around the village, as I'd be sheltered by the houses. This would have meant running the loop nearly thirty-three times! But as the day approached, the early hours looked quite promising, with minimal wind and no rain. So I decided to run a few big loops outside of the village before heading back to finish off the race in the village.

I prepared everything I needed for the race while my son was at school. The next day, I just needed to double-check my gear and decide on my final outfit. I wanted everything to be ready for race day. The weather forecast predicted a temperature of 6 degrees Celsius (real feel), so I opted for a thin vest as a base layer, a technical shirt, long leggings, gloves and a headband to keep my ears warm. I also brought along a light jacket just in case, which I ended up not needing it as the weather was milder than expected.

I woke up early on the Saturday morning and mistakenly thought it was race day. After double-checking the date and my race schedule, I realised my error and went back to sleep. Although it was a momentary lapse in memory, it added a bit of humour to the pre-race jitters, thinking it was race day the day before! Despite the mix-up, I decided to take advantage of the 'extra' day and spend a relaxing day with my family. I spent quality time with my son and husband, trying to distract myself from the upcoming race and enjoy the moment.

In the evening, I spent some time carefully applying kinesiology tape to my knee and the ball of my foot for extra support – probably more than I needed, but I wanted to be sure. With everything in place, I settled in to watch some TV and get some rest before the big day.

On the actual marathon day, I woke up at around 4 am and tried to go back to sleep after having a light breakfast. However, I couldn't fall asleep, so I decided to get ready for my run. I checked the weather one last time and saw it had improved significantly. The wind wasn't as strong as forecasted and there was no rain in sight. I knew that this would make the race much more manageable.

Since it was still dark outside, I put on my headlight and planned to run the first part of my route in the village. After finishing all my pre-run preparations, I did a short warm-up and was ready to start my run. But I couldn't find my gloves. I looked everywhere. I was sure I'd put them out ready for this run, and yet I couldn't find them. I looked in the drawer, in my running bag, and even in my son's school bag, in case he might have taken them for some reason. Finally, after I gave up looking and decided to use a different pair, I spotted them in my dog's mouth. In that moment I was so annoyed; I'd wasted all that time looking for them, and all along my dog had taken a fancy to them. Albeit a bit damp from the dog's slobber, I couldn't resist wearing them for my run.

As I began the race, I felt good. I was running at a steady pace, and my knee and foot were not bothering me. I felt like I was in the zone, and my mind was focused entirely on the task at hand. I was running strong and feeling good.

Even though I don't like running in the dark, I found a way to make it more comfortable. I imagined Stanley running with me: as I ran, I visualised him running alongside me, making me feel safe and content. Though it was just my imagination, the feeling of not being alone was comforting. I repeated to myself that this was just a regular Sunday long run with a medal waiting for me at the end. This helped to ease some of my anxiety and nerves.

After running just over 6 miles, I left the village to do my favourite loop. The wind was far more manageable than it had been for my first marathon, but that wasn't the only reason why this marathon differed greatly from my first one. This time, I was in control of the marathon, whereas during my first one, the marathon controlled me. Whenever my pace began to drop, I pushed myself a bit harder to maintain my goal. At the halfway mark, I saw a local farmer who always encouraged me during my training runs. His support was especially welcome at this point. I felt amazing until I hit 15–16 miles when the wind started to pick up, and I began to feel it was a bit too much for my liking. Although it wasn't too terrible, I was eager to return to the village where the houses would give me protection from the cold wind.

The last 8 miles of my run took place within the village, including a short loop that passed by my son's school (the one I had toyed with running for the entire marathon). Unfortunately, I struggled to remember to take my gels and to drink enough water. Although I took one gel upon arriving in the village, I realised later that I should have taken one more to sustain my energy levels.

As the end drew closer, the physical and mental strain of the marathon was taking its toll. Paul and Jacob had now joined me, cheering me on outside the school as I passed on each loop, which was helpful, but I longed for some extra encouragement. Running alongside someone would have made such a difference for those final miles. With only 6 miles left to go, a group of cyclists passed me. One of them noticed my London Marathon bib and shared the news with the others. Their words of encouragement were just what I needed to push through the remaining distance. I had assumed that more people would have noticed me running with a bib number, but few actually did.

Despite experiencing pain under my foot, I persevered to finish the race. Although I had tried to go faster during the final parts of the race, I didn't have more speed in me. I had worked hard to become faster but couldn't push myself further. Looking back, perhaps I could have made some quicker strides. I picked up the pace slightly, but since there was no designated finish line, it wasn't easy to gauge how much further I had left to run. When my Garmin watch showed I'd reached 26.2 miles, I stopped my watch, only to realise that the London Marathon app had glitched and showed I still had 0.2 miles to run. I continued running, but the app seemed to stall at 26.2 miles, meaning I technically still hadn't finished the marathon. It was a rather confusing ending to the race, but finally I saw I had finished, and I returned home where my husband took photos of my triumph and I could relax.

In the end, my Garmin calculated a finish time of 4 hours and 26 minutes and the London Marathon app stated 4 hours and 29 minutes. I was ecstatic! I had achieved my goal, and it felt amazing. I knew how much hard work, determination, and positive attitude it had taken to get to this point. Meditation and visualisation during the last weeks of my training had been crucial to achieving my goal. I had done it, and I was proud of myself for that.

When I completed the marathon, it didn't quite feel real. Leading up to the race, I was very apprehensive, worried that my injuries would prevent me from running, and I was mentally preparing to walk most of it. I don't think I fully realised what this marathon meant to me. The fact that I was able to complete my second marathon in under 4 hours and 30 minutes just seemed too good to be true.

The Virtual London Marathon was a rollercoaster of emotions, but it turned out to be a great experience for me. It taught me that despite setbacks and injuries, it's important to keep pushing forward and to believe in yourself. It also showed me that with a positive attitude, anything is possible.

Chapter 16:
The Way Forward

The best way to predict the future is to create it.

ABRAHAM LINCOLN

A month after completing the Virtual London Marathon I ran a local 10k race. (We'll come back to that race in part III.) After that, I found myself in a state of uncertainty. Self-doubt crept in yet again as I began comparing myself to other runners and questioned my own status as a 'real runner'.

Although I had another local race (a 10-miler) booked for a few months' time, I wasn't sure what my next steps would be beyond that. I knew I wanted to run a half marathon in the spring and potentially one or two marathons later that year, and maybe train for my first ultra –depending on my ability.

I was still not completely free of injuries, and I kept getting niggles. I did my best to cope with them; as long as I was progressing, even if the progress was slow, I was happy. I had learned a lot from my past injuries, such as the importance of good running form, proper warm-up and cool-down techniques, and when to replace my running shoes. To complement my running and reduce the risk of injury, I also started taking swimming lessons.

I have a deep love for running, but being prone to injury means that I must accept my limitations and find an exercise routine that complements my running. Although I had swimming lessons as a child, I never became a confident swimmer and was always afraid of deep water. Open water swimming is common in Estonia; designated swimming spots are located throughout the country, making it easy to find a safe and convenient swimming location. As a child, I was never as brave as my sister or her friends, who would swim across the lakes and rivers while I clung to the edge. I always felt embarrassed because it seemed that swimming was a skill that everyone had. As an adult, I made several attempts to learn proper swimming techniques, but only made it to a few lessons. Now, eight years after my last attempt, I was giving it another go. I was determined to overcome my fear of deep water.

As I mastered the proper techniques of swimming and even enjoyed it, I found pleasure in the learning process. We rented a local swimming pool as a family and each time we went swimming together I vowed we'd make it a regular activity. But, life gets in the way, and, regrettably, swimming just doesn't evoke the same passion within me as running does. I've since decided I'll stick with activities that I enjoy more.

With one defeat conquered I knew that I could overcome another fear of mine. I really wanted to run a 100-mile race, but one thing was holding me back: it requires running through the night, in the dark. I am afraid of the dark. Since childhood I have struggled with darkness and this was definitely not going to be an easy fear to overcome. Running 100 miles seemed an impossible feat, but something drew me to this challenge. I knew it would take many months to prepare, and the challenge would consume my life, but I still found the distance incredibly alluring. Conquering my fear of swimming gave me hope that maybe I could overcome my fear of darkness too…

A bigger barrier, however, was that my running wasn't going as I wanted it to. I used to be very determined and never walked during a run, thinking that real runners would never walk. Although I'd heard of the run/walk method and knew many runners used it, I didn't want to. In time, I would appreciate the need and value of walking during a run, but at this point I found myself wanting to give up during runs and losing confidence in my abilities. I knew part of it was post-marathon blues, but I just couldn't bounce back this time around. I was still running, but it felt a bit 'meh'. It was like I just wasn't bothered.

During my next long run I wanted to cover the half marathon distance: I knew it would boost my confidence. My goal for the run wasn't to achieve a fast time, but to finish the distance, no matter how slow it may be. Target set, I began. My progress was good until around the 8k (5-mile) mark, when I began to feel pain in my knee. A negative inner dialogue immediately started, as I started thinking about how uncomfortable the pain was and how strong the wind was. I considered stopping and going home to sulk on the sofa instead of continuing my run.

However, I caught myself and decided to change my thinking. I started telling myself that my knees were strong and that I was enjoying the run; I reminded myself how much I had missed my Sunday morning runs and that it was great to be out running again. By changing my mindset, I began to push through the pain (which soon disappeared!) and complete the run. Getting to the finish line of this half marathon distance gave me a huge boost and helped restore some of my confidence in running.

I still had my huge goal in mind, but I realised I'd need to break it down into smaller goals. My running game and motivation improved suddenly after chatting with Becky in the running club. She mentioned a race called Dukeries 30/40, which she'd done for her thirtieth birthday. I'd somehow missed this one in my search for the perfect first ultra. The event takes place in May each year in the stunning Sherwood Forest, and features a 30.8-mile or 40.8-mile route. The upcoming race only offered the 40-mile option, which was perfect for me. I loved the idea that the event organisers exclusively offer vegan food at aid stations. As a plant-based participant, the availability of vegan options provided me with peace of mind and took away any worries about consuming animal products.

Despite my past injuries in the back of my mind, I was eager to sign up for an ultra and believed that I could get to the finish line. Although I was a little apprehensive, running an ultra had been a strong ambition of mine since before even completing my first marathon. With a change in my training routines and feeling better about my running, I was now more determined than ever to set new goals for myself. I knew that achieving my longer-term goal of running a 100-miler would take time, effort, and dedication, and I was willing to put in the work to make it happen. But first: the 40-miler!

One of the first things I focused on was building my confidence in my running abilities. I had let injuries and setbacks get the better of me in the past, but I knew I could do so much more. I worked on visualising my goals and focusing on the positive aspects of my runs rather than dwelling on the negative.

I also continued to work on my running form and technique, which I'd picked up during my running coach training. Good form was vital to avoid injuries and maximise performance; learning and implementing new exercises and drills would improve my form and make me a stronger runner. Additionally, I worked on incorporating the right strength and conditioning exercises into my training routine. In the past, my strength training routine was dictated mostly by my various niggles and injuries. Now, I was able to focus on general strength building for running. I complemented my running with cross-training such as cycling and yoga to make me a well-rounded athlete.

Throughout it all, I never gave up on my dreams. I knew that there would be times when training would be hard and there would be setbacks along the way. But I remembered why I started running in the first place and kept pushing forward. I reminded myself that anything was possible if I was willing to work for it. With determination, hard work, and a positive attitude, I knew that I could achieve my goals and become the best runner I could be.

Chapter 17:
Forced Running Break

*If you don't pick a day to relax,
your body will pick it for you.*

Unknown

It has been a month since my last run, and I'm struggling to find the motivation to get back into it. I've never had problems with motivation in the past, but this time feels different. I've been dealing with a cold that turned into a sinus and chest infection, and the time off running has taken its toll on my fitness and mental state. Physical injury in the past was easier to cope with, as I was still able to cross-train. Having an illness just made me feel that I should have tried harder.

This morning, I reached out to my WhatsApp running group to see if anyone wanted to join me for a run – secretly hoping that no one would be available so that I could cancel. After my Virtual London Marathon I started a small running group in my village (more about this later in chapter 28, 'Running Group'). But when multiple responses came in from people unable to make it, I was surprised to feel a rush of disappointment.

When I first noticed a tickle in my throat a month before, I didn't pay much attention to it. I have had colds before; I usually skip a few runs, and am soon back to it. This time it felt different. My cold seemed to improve slightly, only to worsen again. The cough was the worst part. After a weekend with earache and sinus pain, I called my GP. It turned out I had bacterial sinusitis and a chest infection. After a week on antibiotics, I was still not convinced about my ability to run.

The constant coughing had also aggravated my incontinence issues, which had been under control for a while and didn't impact my running any more. It was disheartening to feel embarrassed and depressed, and I just generally felt exhausted. I was altogether feeling unsure about everything to do with running, including my ability to continue leading the running group sessions and connecting with other runners. While I was happy about their progress, I couldn't help but feel stuck and frustrated with my own lack of progress. I was uncertain about what to do next. Above all though, I knew by this point what a difference a change in mindset can make when it comes to change.

I'd signed up for my first ultra before I got ill; I knew I had to stop sulking and get back to running. The first step towards change is often the hardest one to take, but I firmly believe that I have the strength and ability to make a positive change in my life, even when feeling down about myself and everything else. I had recently taken a step towards that change by trying to run as a way to improve my mood rather than focusing on distance or worrying about any races I had coming up. I didn't even bother changing my clothes; I hopped on the treadmill and gave it a shot.

Even though I know the walk/run method works for many people, I struggle, even now, with 'allowing' myself to do it. I decided to give it a try and ran for 2.5 minutes, then walked for 30 seconds. I repeated this for about 15 minutes and started to feel better. Physically, I could have kept going, but the monotony of the treadmill wasn't enough to motivate me to continue.

The following morning, I woke up early and managed to fit in a short strength training routine before meeting up with my friend Laura for a planned run. The strength training session felt challenging, but I knew it was necessary after taking a break from it for over a month. However, just as I prepared to head out for the run, I felt my knee tense. *Not again!* I thought. I was frustrated and discouraged: although I knew my niggles were now a part of my running, I didn't want to risk making things worse. Even so, I had committed to my friend and didn't want to let her down.

We ran for a few minutes and then did some warm-up exercises and dynamic stretches – I had almost forgotten my warm-up routine! Then we started running again, but it just felt so hard. And my knee was still hurting. We looked at each other and said, 'Shall we walk?'

When we eased to a walk, I felt how my pain was going. We continued with these run/walk intervals for nearly 6.5k. At some point, I noticed my pain was completely gone. I think it was just my brain messing with me. That run made such a difference to my attitude towards running. Before this run, although I knew it was perfectly okay to walk during the runs, I would still beat myself up if I ever needed to walk. Doing a run/walk with a dear friend helped me to become kinder to myself.

The night before, I had been in a negative headspace, regretting my decision to take time off running and feeling like I had lost my progress. But this run reminded me that progress isn't always linear and that it's important to be patient with myself. After such setbacks, I know it will take time to rebuild my strength and confidence, but I also know I can get there.

Injury may restrict you from running but instead you can cross-train or engage in other activities. Physical illness is entirely different from injury and can make it challenging to perform any activity at all. Even getting through the day and completing routine tasks, such as walking the dog or caring for one's family, can be difficult. It's important to recognise that both physical illness and injury can be challenging to cope with, and seeking support from healthcare professionals, family, and friends can make a big difference. While the experience of physical illness can be overwhelming, it's important to focus on small accomplishments and celebrate even the smallest victories.

One thing I learned from this forced running break is the importance of patience and self-compassion. I can't expect to jump back into my previous running routine and performance without giving my body the time and care it needs to heal and recover. I valued the importance of listening to my body and not pushing myself too hard, too soon.

When you're feeling down, it's vital to focus on one thing at a time. Sometimes it's best to give yourself a break and skip an evening run, curling up on the sofa with your favourite drink and watching TV or reading a book instead. Other times, you have to put on your big girl pants and push through the discomfort. Just go out for a run. Rarely have I regretted a run after completing it. Whether you need to take a break or push yourself forward, remember to focus on the present moment and take things one step at a time (sometimes literally!).

My goal to run my first ultra became the main driving force behind wanting to break through the injury/illness cycle that was plaguing me. I needed to get better to achieve my goal!

Chapter 18:
Run the Thames

*Medals may not make the runners,
but they sure make us feel good about our run.*

UNKNOWN

After a setback from being ill for a month at the end of the year, I needed a challenge at the start of the following year that would push me back on track. That's when I came across the virtual 'Run the Thames' race, where you had to run or walk 214 miles between 1 January and 21 February. The challenge comes with a beautiful medal that I'd admired the previous year but felt too exhausted from the heavier mileage required for the Land's End to John o'Groats challenge I'd just completed (the injury I sustained soon after meant I wouldn't have been able to complete it anyway). I'd been eagerly looking forward to hanging the Thames medal on my medal rack ever since.

This time, I was excited set myself a daring goal and push myself to complete the 214 miles. Even though the distance felt daunting, achieving such a feat and the reward of the medal would make it all worthwhile. I also saw this as the perfect start for my ultra training. Completing Run the Thames required me to run around 29 miles a week. This is not much in the middle of marathon training but can be pretty demanding when you're just building up your fitness. After losing so much fitness from being poorly, I needed some sort of test that would push me back on track. I looked forward to the challenge and the personal success that would come from completing it.

On New Year's Day, I had a stomach bug, but I still went for a run. I decided to keep it short, just running in the village so I would be close enough to get to home on time if I needed to use the toilet. Surprisingly, I didn't need to and ran 4 enjoyable miles that day.

I attempted to run a bit further during that first week of January. When I had to pick up some clothes in a nearby village I decided to run, instead of taking the car. The weather was decent, so I took an empty backpack to put the clothes in and headed out. I felt good to start with, and I got to my destination feeling great. Getting back home was a different story. I began to feel tired, and home seemed so far away. I considered calling Paul and seeing if he'd pick me up, but it seemed silly. I wanted to be strong and carry on; I didn't want to walk. I was afraid that if I started walking, I wouldn't get back to my running stride.

So I reminded myself of my mantra, 'I own this run', and focused on the next nominal landmark: the next tree, the next row of hedges, the houses in the distance. I realised that if I just focused on the next few hundred metres at a time, I could make it. Slowly, I started to get closer to home. When I reached the village, I turned my music back on, and the last mile didn't feel that bad at all. When I got home and sat down, my husband jokingly told our son that Mummy had just run a marathon. It was only 10 miles, but it felt like a marathon in that moment.

Over the following weeks, I tried to forget how slow I had become during the forced break from running and concentrated on getting the miles in, however slow they were. Gradually, I started to get faster. It was a faster mile here or there, which then turned into a few more. I wasn't doing any speed training during this period; I just wanted to become friends with running again.

Then came the day when I decided to run 10 miles to meet my weekly goal for the challenge. In the time since my victorious 10 miles to the village I had run a few 8-mile loops, but most of my runs were on the shorter side. On the day of my 10-mile challenge it felt hard, as it sometimes does at the beginning of a long run. I reminded myself it would get easier as the run progressed and this helped me to push forward. Somewhere before the 10-mile mark, I decided to go further instead of returning. I originally planned to get an extra mile in, but then I just kept running and thought I would try to run 13 miles. Running a half marathon has always been some sort of landmark for me. It doesn't matter how fast or slow it is: after that my running seems to get back on track.

At some point during my run, I felt like it was getting tough. I initially thought it was because of the distance, but then I realised I was running a lot faster than I had during the first part of my run. Slowing down to conserve energy crossed my mind, but running that little bit faster felt so natural, like it was exactly what I was meant to do. As I continued, I hit a point where it became mentally challenging. I wasn't physically tired, but I found myself getting bored and craving some kind of distraction. I briefly considered calling Paul and asking him to get me, but I knew that would mean a long round trip for him. So instead, I decided to focus on seemingly inconsequential landmarks and just keep pushing myself.

As I got closer to home, I kept running, focusing on the road ahead, 300–400 metres at a time. Before I knew it, I had completed the half marathon distance, plus a bit more! It had been nearly three months since I'd last run a half marathon. I felt such gratification and pride as I finished the distance, urging myself to run further than I had planned. I experienced a great sense of gratitude once again as I overcame my fears and limitations and ran a longer distance.

The following week, this elating long run was replaced with a sudden lack of motivation to run. A lot seemed to be going on in my life, and I couldn't shake off the anxiety. On the Monday, I put on my running gear in the morning, thinking that I would head out for a run after dropping my son off at school and walking the dog. When I returned from walking the dog, however, I felt so cold that I didn't feel like going out for a run any more. Instead, I decided to use the treadmill. I had planned to do an easy 30-minute run to at least get some mileage in. I stopped after just 10 minutes. It felt so dull and pointless.

The next day was a running group day: we were going to practise for the running coach assessment day that was coming up the following weekend. I delivered the session and went out for a short run to add to my mileage. When I got home, I saw that I had seventy-three messages in the running coach WhatsApp group. As I briefly scrolled through the messages, I saw that some people couldn't do the assessment on Saturday as one of the assessors was no longer available. There was uncertainty about who was able to do the assessment and who wasn't. With that added worry, the house in a mess and the dog needing to be walked, I decided to focus on those tasks instead.

Unfortunately, the rest of the Run the Thames race did not go as expected, and I struggled to accumulate enough running miles. During a family holiday in February I tried to run as much as I could, but ended up doing more walking than running. My dream of completing the challenge with running miles alone started slipping away. Rather than give up completely, I ran as much as my schedule allowed, and (as a last resort) I added some walking miles to achieve the total and receive the medal.

Despite the setbacks, I achieved my primary objective, which was to run more frequently, regain consistency in my running routine, and get in as many miles as possible.

Throughout the challenge, I learned that it's essential to not only set goals but to also be flexible with them. I also respected the importance of consistency. Even on days when I didn't feel like running, I made sure to get out there and put in the miles.

Over time, this helped me to build up my stamina and speed gradually.

Above all, the virtual Run the Thames challenge helped me to get back on track with my running and reignite my passion for the sport, at a time when I felt utterly defeated and lacked any sort of motivation.

Chapter 19:
Forty Miles for My 40th

If you want to run, run a mile.
If you want to experience a different life, run a marathon.
If you want to talk to God, run an ultra.

DEAN KARNAZES

Ultra running shows how things that once seemed impossible can become possible. This book started out with a compulsion to write about my running experience from zero to marathon (whether that be a blog post or a letter to a running magazine). At the time, the prospect of running a marathon seemed an impossible task, but when I achieved it, I believed that only more positive results lay ahead. However, much like life itself, running is subject to highs and lows. I had to learn how to cope with extended periods of injury, how to manage both physical and emotional struggles such as depression and incontinence, and how to recover my footing after bouts of sickness.

When writing this chapter, I was in training for my very first ultra marathon, Dukeries 40, a challenge I never even imagined taking on just a year and a half ago. While I was thrilled to be preparing for this race, I was aware that the coming months would present their own set of difficulties. However, 2021 taught me a great deal about perseverance and making my aspirations happen, even when progress seemed sluggish.

At the start of 2022, I hoped to be highly motivated and to do some great running. Run the Thames gave me a head start, but then, almost out of nowhere, I felt down again and not motivated to run. Whenever I had an excuse good enough, I would skip my runs. This continued until I realised that I only had twelve weeks left to train for a 40.8-mile race. I had written my ultra race training plan months ago, but it looked bare and incomplete due to a lack of structured running. Although I was still running, my distance and frequency were not what I had planned. I had to adjust my plans to fit where I had managed to get to.

For my ultra training, I created a plan based on the ones I'd used for my two marathons. This included a few back-to-back runs and plenty of cross-training in the form of cycling. The principle is still the same: three key runs during the week, comprising an interval session, a tempo run, and a long run. In addition, I did two cycling sessions and two strength training sessions a week. I also continued to plan and deliver running group sessions. Sometimes I did my interval session after running with the group, sometimes the next day.

After following my training plan for two weeks I felt good. I had to put much faith into listening to my body and hoping my training plan would work. Most ultra training plans suggested running more, but I had to be smart here. As much as I wanted to get to the finish line, I needed to make it to the start line first. I was also still struggling with the persistent pain under my foot that first occurred in the end of 2020, despite numerous visits to the podiatrist and physiotherapist. However, I had come to accept that this injury would always be there, and my focus shifted to managing it in such a way that it didn't hinder my running too much.

Running during the first lockdown felt easy. Perhaps I was looking at it through rose-tinted glasses or maybe it was because my progress was linear. I was getting faster every few weeks, building my distance, and generally improving. However, after my injuries and illness in 2021, my progress seemed to be one step forward and two steps back. Although, for the most part, I kept running through the injuries (during the illness, I had to stop altogether), I wasn't able to progress as I wanted to because my ability to train was always dictated by my pain. I felt that if I had been able to be consistent with my training, I would have been able to make some real progress with my running.

Ten weeks before the Dukeries race, I got an appointment with an NHS physio after waiting for nineteen weeks. 'Why now?', you might ask. Although I was able to run and follow my training plans for the most part, in addition to my foot pain, I knew my left knee was still my weak spot, and I didn't want it to put an end to my ultra dreams. The goal of this appointment was to sort my body out once and for all. By the time of my appointment, I had something new – a pain in my hip.

I didn't have high hopes for that appointment. My previous experiences with my physio appointments at the sports physio clinic for my IT band injury hadn't really provided me with the help I was hoping for.

This physiotherapist was a tall man in his sixties. He called me in and asked me to sit on the examination bed. 'What brings you here today?' he asked in a kind voice.

'There's something wrong with my left side. I started running during the lockdown, and despite things going well in the beginning, I keep getting injured,' I answered. I talked about my long recovery from ITBS and mentioned that I still experienced knee pain on and off and how I have to replace running with cycling when that happens. I also mentioned the pain under the ball of my foot and the new hip pain (although it had eased slightly by the time of the appointment).

He asked me to lie on the examination bed, and he moved my knee in different directions to identify any limitations or discomfort. Then, he instructed me to perform single-leg squats as part of his assessment. Although I regularly did these, it felt odd doing them while being evaluated. He examined my knee once more, and I anxiously awaited his verdict. I was afraid that he wouldn't really understand how important running is to me and might suggest that I run less, forgetting about my ultra dream. Instead, it seemed like the stars had aligned just right: he was actually a runner himself.

He said that my left knee was not correctly aligned and I needed to strengthen the muscles around my knee. My left side had always seemed weaker and all my problems were anchored there: it all made sense now. He only gave me two exercises to do, but I had to do those three times a day. For my IT band he showed me a beautiful (but ever so painful) stretch. I still use it often, especially before and after long runs. There was no fancy massage or nice pink kinesiology tape like at the sports physio clinic that I visited before. Even my exercises were just scribbled on a piece of paper instead of detailed plans with YouTube videos that the clinic provided. Still, I was full of hope that this time things would improve for good.

For my foot pain, he just recommended that I get cushier trainers. In regards to my hip issue, he diagnosed it as bursitis, which I should be able to easily alleviate with some rest, icing, and massaging using a spiky ball (once it felt better). It was very effective but quite painful. This was when I wondered if it might be time to invest in an actual foam roller instead.

The physio exercises were extremely helpful and made me feel like I was on the right track towards permanent recovery; I could feel the difference when I trained. Two weeks after seeing the physio I ran a 16-mile off-road training run, during which I was delighted (and surprised) to feel no pain in the ball of my foot. It was a good start for me. I also discovered that I really enjoyed off-road running, which I hadn't done much of since my recovery period after my first marathon. I loved being in tune with the ground and my surroundings, and the distance seemed less significant. Although I ran slower, the time seemed to fly by.

That year the Easter school holidays were a week longer than usual, but my progress remained unbroken. I began doing back-to-back runs, completing them successfully, including a 21-mile run one day and 12 miles the next. It felt easy, and I felt unstoppable on my path towards the Dukeries race. The final week of the holidays was a struggle for me to get out for a run, however. I couldn't go in the mornings due to my husband leaving for work early and I felt too tired in the evenings. I had my first paid coaching session planned for the weekend and decided to run only a short distance before that. On the day of the session, however, my client cancelled due to being stuck on a train. While I understood it wasn't her fault, I couldn't help but feel disappointed. Later that day, I went for a run but felt hot and bothered, and my headphones didn't connect properly. I managed to get some mileage in but less than planned, so I added some time on the indoor bike to make up for it.

The following week, I had two new coaching clients and had to prepare for my son's birthday party. With Paul getting poorly and unable to help me with the party, my time became very limited. The week after that, I had an appointment with a podiatrist who prescribed new insoles to try to ease the pain under the ball of my foot, which was still coming and going. I had hoped this would be a magic cure for the stubborn pain under my foot, which affected me most during my road runs. However, after wearing them for only half a day, my ankle began to hurt. It could have just been a coincidence, but my ankle continued to hurt even after several days of rest. In hindsight, it could have been just a result of increasing my distance and running off-road more often. I tried taping it up and running on it, as my motivation to run had returned, but the pain persisted. In the end, I decided to book an appointment for a few days' time with the physio who had helped with my knee pain.

The physio listened to my symptoms and bluntly said that I wouldn't be able to run an ultra. Seeing my face fall, he shared his experience of being injured while training for the London Marathon and having to replace running with cycling, yet still achieving a very good time. This gave me hope. He said that I would probably be able to run bits of my ultra and walk some. In the meantime, he recommended that I avoid running altogether and suggested indoor cycling instead. I took his advice and cycled religiously for the next few weeks.

When my ankle began to feel better, I took my rides outside, still unable to run. I completed a difficult cycling session, mimicking my longest run before the ultra. I pushed myself to the limit, cycling on the hardest gear for speed; it was tough and my legs ached, but I pushed through. It proved to be good mental preparation for the ultra. Gradually, I added short runs to my cycling routine, adjusting to the feeling of running again after a long hiatus. These brief runs helped me prepare mentally for the race, as I felt that I couldn't significantly influence my physical performance at that stage. A week before the race my longest run was now only 5 miles. My last proper long run was now six weeks ago, which felt like ages ago, but I still had faith I could do it. Recalling the physio's experience with the London Marathon gave me hope.

As the days leading up to the Dukeries ultra dwindled down, I felt a mixture of excitement and nerves. I turned my attention to my fuelling plan for the day and what I'd put in my race pack. Fuelling for an ultra was uncharted territory for me. I knew how to get through a marathon, but anything beyond that was guesswork. I had steered away from gels and mainly used baby food pouches during my long runs, but I knew that wouldn't be enough for a 40.8-mile race. Whenever I researched and asked other ultra runners for advice, the answer was always the same: what works for one person might not work for another.

Ultimately, I decided to pack the foods I knew worked for me and rely on aid stations for the rest. I planned to listen to my body and give it what it craved. Experienced ultra runners recommended eating often and well before feeling hungry, so I planned to have a little bit of something every 30 minutes. My fuel plan included two flavours of baby food fruit pouches, some gels, salt tablets for electrolytes, and dried mango. I was hesitant about adding the dried mango, which I had never used during runs before, but I wanted a sweet treat that I loved. In the days leading up to the race, I ate normally but found myself craving mango ice cream, which I made from bananas, frozen mango, and soya milk. I decided to give my body what it wanted and not stress too much about it.

To stay hydrated, I packed my trusty water bladder and salt tablets. I carefully packed and unpacked my race pack multiple times, mindful of the weight. In addition to fuel, I packed essentials such as a battery pack for my phone, headphones, paper maps (in case I got lost), Vaseline (I didn't have a small enough container for my usual nappy cream), and a waterproof jacket. I used most of the items I brought, but the first aid kit, jacket, and paper maps remained untouched. However, I felt reassured knowing that they were there in case of an emergency.

    I had put in the hard work, faced my fair share of setbacks, and now it was time to put my training to the test. Mentally, I felt ready to tackle the 40 miles ahead of me. Physically, I knew I had done everything in my power to prepare. I focused on getting plenty of rest, staying hydrated, and sticking to my nutrition plan.

Chapter 20:
Dukeries

A runner must run with dreams in his heart.

Emil Zatopek

I'm going to run over 40 miles tomorrow, I thought, feeling overwhelmed by the distance. It seemed impossibly far, and while I was excited, I was also anxious. I went to bed early but struggled to fall asleep. I had spent the week leading up to my first ultra marathon reading and preparing. Though my preparation wasn't perfect, I had researched how to cope with the 'pain cave' and watched videos of others running similar distances. To distract myself from the upcoming challenge, I continued reading the book on my nightstand – Adharanand Finn's *The Rise of the Ultra Runners*. It's a great book, and concentrating on something other than my racing thoughts was a welcome change.

When I woke up at 3 am on race day, I felt at peace with myself and ready to tackle the challenge ahead. I felt happy. I was fortunate enough to get a lift with some seasoned ultra runners who had done the route before, which helped to calm my nerves. On arrival, everything went smoothly: we collected our numbers, visited the toilets, and posed for the group photo. I started to do my warm-up exercises, and then it was already time for the race brief.

As I stood at the starting line, surrounded by other determined runners, I couldn't help but feel proud of how far I had come. The journey had taken me through injuries, personal loss, and many hard running miles, but I had learned a lot about myself along the way: mainly the power of perseverance and the importance of taking care of both my mind and body. I was determined to cross the finish line, and no matter the outcome, I knew that I would never forget this experience.

When Ronnie, the race director, announced during the race briefing that a diversion was in place to avoid the flood, I felt relieved. Almost every year, there is a section on the route early on where runners have to wade through water for about 100 metres and I really didn't want to get my feet wet. I had mentally prepared myself to cope with it if I had to, but thankfully, I wouldn't need to. Things were going well so far.

Ronnie asked, 'Are there people running the Robin Hood 100 in September, too?' before adding, 'This race is a good recce for it.' After hearing this, I instantly knew this was the 100-mile race I'd been looking for; the one the Dukeries was a taster for.

I whispered to Hannah, who was standing next to me, 'I'd like to run that race in the future.'

'Go for it!' Hannah replied. I had read the race descriptions for that event while preparing for Dukeries, and it had been on my mind for a while, but it felt scary to admit it to someone; it just seemed like too big of a goal to set. How could I decide I wanted to run 100 miles without running an ultra race first? I suppose it was the same with my first ultra. I knew I wanted to run an ultra race even before I'd completed my first marathon.

There was another lady, Caroline, from my running club who planned to run the Dukeries at a similar pace as me. At first, I was glad to have the company, so we started together. However, after a few miles, I realised it wasn't really working for me. I had never run with her before and kept trying to match her stride; I missed my own music and my own thoughts and I wasn't enjoying it. I had trained alone, and I knew I needed to run alone. So, I let her go and put on my music, instantly feeling free and able to run at my own pace.

I was worried about my ankle and the lack of running in the weeks leading up to the ultra. I found the running quite challenging in the early stages, but I was hopeful that it would improve as I got more miles under my belt. And, in a way, it did improve. I distinctly remember arriving at the second aid station and feeling like I had a spring in my step – I was feeling really good. I grabbed a banana to have later and continued on my way. I had promised to let my husband know when I was passing the aid stations, but unfortunately I had no reception on my phone. I tried to message him after passing The Major Oak (a 1,000-year-old oak tree in Sherwood Forest, supposedly the hideout of Robin Hood) because he was planning to come and see it later that day with our son, but still no luck. I kept trying to send messages periodically, but nothing went through. I was annoyed but just tried to let the feeling go. All I could do was keep running.

I met several people on the route and ran short sections with them. There was a couple running the race at a similar overall pace as me. We must have passed each other thirty times or so. It kept my spirits up and put a smile to my face, and I felt like I always had someone nearby.

As I approached the aid stations, I reminded myself to keep my pit stops short and efficient. I grabbed what I needed and continued moving forward, even if it meant eating on the go. Luckily, I found that the jam sandwiches and watermelon provided by the aid stations were a perfect addition to my own snacks. The sweet and juicy flavours were a welcome treat and helped to keep my energy levels up as I pushed through the gruelling miles. I was grateful for the aid station volunteers who made sure that these options, alongside many others, were available, as they provided a much-needed boost when I needed it most.

When I felt that running was too much, I walked. But I was always moving, whether running or walking. I looked at my watch and saw that the time was ticking away, so I pushed myself to run again, and I just kept running. I knew that there would be challenges ahead, but I was determined to finish this race.

I was heading to the last aid station. There were 11 miles between this aid station and the previous one. As I arrived at the final station I felt like there wasn't much more distance left to cover to get to the end. I can't thank the volunteers enough in that aid station. Since my phone wasn't working, I asked one of the marshals if I could use his phone and managed to text Paul. It was a relief to know that my husband knew I was okay, though I was still a bit worried about him not knowing where I was along the route. When I asked him later about it, he reassured me that he knew I was okay in his heart and he hadn't worried about me.

As I continued on my way, I spotted some cows in the distance. I desperately hoped I could avoid them as for some reason I am afraid of these animals. However, I soon realised that the path went directly through the field they were in. I glanced around, hoping to find an alternative route. Nope, there wasn't one. Feeling panicked, I realised I had no choice but to go through them. Eventually, I gathered my courage and proceeded forward at a slow and steady pace. Once safely past them, I picked up my pace, eager to leave the field behind as quickly as possible.

Other than those cows, I had been running alone for a while and wondered where everyone had gone. Then, I suddenly saw someone far ahead waving to me. At first, I thought it was a volunteer showing us the way, but it turned out to be Sarah from the running club! I was so happy to see her. She wasn't running the ultra; she was there supporting her husband who had already finished. It had been a long time since I'd had contact with anyone I already knew before the race, and it gave me a significant boost. She ran with me for a bit and promised to join me again. She also said she'd contact Paul and let him know how I was doing.

I found myself walking more than I had anticipated during the later stages of the race. It was a strange feeling because I always say to others it's okay to walk during a run, but I felt ashamed taking the same advice myself. But the truth was that my body was tired, and walking was necessary to conserve energy and push through the remaining miles. I also struggled to understand how much distance I had left to run. As I usually run in kilometres, I had memorised the distance in miles between all the aid stations. However, with route diversions and me taking a wrong turn, I just wasn't sure how much exactly was left.

As I got closer to the finish line, I wanted to run more. But rather than feeling a rush of adrenaline propelling me forward, I felt a wave of calm wash over me as the relief of knowing the end was so close flowed through me. I had accomplished what I set out to do; all that was left was finishing the final stretch. The strange thing was that I was physically capable of running, and I ran sections between walking. But walking just seemed so much more comfortable and easier at that moment. So I walked for a while longer, taking in the sights and sounds around me.

The finish can't be far now, let's run this last bit! I told myself, as I dragged my heavy legs back to running.

I'd watched videos about the finish line and visualised it so many times during my preparation. There aren't big crowds waiting for you, but there are people who love and care about you, and that's all that matters. As I approached the finish line, I could see the Caistor Running Club members waving a flag and cheering for me. They handed me the Lincolnshire flag, and I felt so honoured to run the final stretch with it. When I crossed the finish line, I felt a sense of victory and utter pride. It was a special moment, and suddenly, I was overwhelmed with emotions. I realised that I had reached my goal – I had finished my first ultra. I was exhausted, but simultaneously, I felt a sense of satisfaction that I had never experienced before. After feeling lonely multiple times during the race, it felt great to finally be able to hug my son and husband.

The joy of finishing didn't last long for me, however. Although I'd completed the race, I felt empty and slightly disappointed that I didn't achieve my goal time of under 8 hours. Nevertheless, I promised myself to come back and beat my time. After cheering on other runners at the finish line, I collected my medal, shirt, and hot soup before finding a place to sit down and savour the warmth of the soup.

As we made our way back to the car and exchanged congratulations with fellow participants, it wasn't until later that night that I could relax on the couch and reflect on what I'd achieved. I couldn't shake this sense of emptiness that lingered within me. I was expecting some sort of epiphany, but I wasn't even in as much pain as I'd assumed I'd be. In the end, I felt like the race didn't seem insurmountable or too challenging and I just didn't reach any sort of euphoria about it.

The first time I truly felt the magnitude of my feat was on the following Monday. As I took my son to school, another parent who knew I had completed the race asked about it, and I showed them a video of my finish. Once again, I was overcome with emotion. My heart now swelled with pride and joy, overshadowing my initial disappointment.

A few weeks after the race, I saw the physio for a follow-up. Yes, the same guy who originally said I wouldn't be able to race.

When he congratulated me on my achievement, it hit me: I had run my first ultra, over 40 miles, and that was truly awesome. Despite the ankle injury I sustained a few weeks before the race interfering with my training plan, I still did it! I had pushed myself to the limit, both physically and mentally, and I had come out on top. A few years prior I couldn't even imagine running more than 5k, but now I had completed an ultra. It was an experience that I would never forget.

The idea of running a 100-mile race had been on my mind during my Dukeries training, but hearing the Robin Hood 100 mentioned during the race brief made it seem more real. However, it didn't become a persistent thought until after I'd finished my first ultra. The more I researched it, the more determined I became to pursue this challenge. I started by volunteering at the 2022 race so I could get more of a feel of the extent of the endurance of the event. I plan to be at the starting line in September 2024.

Here's to chasing my next big dream!

PART III:
MY RUNNING STYLE

Great to still have you with me. The next part of the book was drafted during my long runs, recording the ideas on my phone or penning the ideas down when I'd finished running and got home. Don't expect a linear timeline from these pages – chronological order takes a back seat here. Just join me on some of my runs and thoughts. I hope you find as much enjoyment in reading this part as I did writing it.

Chapter 21:
Running Three Times a Week

The most important day in any running program is rest.

HAL HIGDON

Being a member of several running groups on Facebook, I have found it fascinating to read about other runners' experiences and to offer and receive advice when needed. As a beginner, these groups were an invaluable resource for me.

Despite the importance of rest days in a runner's training routine, I've noticed that some runners view them as taboo. Many running groups advocate running at least five times a week to complete any distance successfully. As someone who only runs three times a week, I've sometimes felt like I'm not a 'real' runner in comparison. But I am simply not able to schedule more running time in my week. As a mother of a young child, it's common to feel a sense of guilt when prioritising exercise or personal time. It can be challenging to balance one's own needs with the needs of their child, particularly when it means spending time apart. However, I often remind myself that taking care of my physical and mental well-being and pursuing my passions can positively impact my son.

Since running five to six times a week did not fit my schedule, I had to explore other options. I found a half marathon training plan that required running three days a week and cross-training for two additional days. I began to follow the principle of running three times a week and adding other activities, such as cycling, to my routine. Occasionally, I would divide one of my sessions into two and run four days a week, but this was rare. Eventually, I discovered that running three times a week and cross-training twice a week was the best approach for my body.

I rarely run less than 10k per session; occasionally I replace my running sessions with either indoor or outdoor cycling especially if I am injured. As a general guideline, I cycle for the same length of time as I would have run – anywhere from 1 to 3 hours per session, depending on how much time I have – and maintain the same intensity level. So an easy run becomes an easy cycle; a tempo run means a tempo pace whilst cycling. Although I don't always manage to cross-train for an additional two days, I aim to stay active through other means, such as taking my dog for daily walks and choosing to walk, run, or cycle instead of driving whenever feasible.

Initially, I did some strength training after each of my three runs. Later, I played around with this a bit and tried incorporating yoga and Pilates into my routine. I found that little and often works better for me than long exercise sessions. I would rather do a daily, short (up to 30 minutes) strength routine rather than an hour at a time, three times a week. I also focus on a good warm-up and cool-down before and after my runs.

At times, fitting in three running sessions a week has been difficult, especially during lockdowns, self-isolation, and school holidays. I plan my activities on the Sunday before, adapting my training plans to accommodate other obligations, though I try to stick to specific days each week for my runs. Other activities, such as cycling, yoga and strength training, I fit in when I can. Over the course of my running journey, I have learned to make time for exercise. Before my son started school I often did my strength and stability work between playing with him and doing chores around the house. I might fold some laundry, do a few reps, play with my son, and then do some more reps. It was challenging to schedule my runs around my son's limited preschool hours, but I still managed to make it work.

After reading Jo Pavey's book *This Mum Runs* and discovering that she used a similar approach to her training, I stopped feeling guilty about it. What matters is getting the necessary training and strength and stability work in, regardless of how it's done. If an Olympian can achieve success with this strategy, it's also acceptable to me. The key is to be adaptable while also prioritising yourself and your fitness at times.

My average week now consists of three runs and three strength training sessions. I do two shorter runs during the week and a long run on the weekend, usually on Sundays. These days I mostly run in the mornings after taking my son to school, but if that's not possible, I run when I can fit it in – early mornings or late evenings. School holidays are challenging, but somehow

I make it work. I might set up a craft table for my son while I am on the exercise bike in the shed. This way, I can still interact with him while doing my exercise at the same time. During the weekends, if I don't have time for a long run and a dog walk, then I just change my session to a canicross session and still get my training done. It is different than running on my own, as it's my dog's run too, but it still counts. Strength training is something I just slot in when there's chance. I might do it in the morning before my son wakes up, or if that's not possible, I sometimes do it during the evening. All of it has had a really positive effect, sparking my son's interest in exercise. Occasionally, he joins in with my strength training routine and is ever so proud of his exercising. (And so am I!)

Despite the popular belief that running a marathon requires a rigorous training schedule of daily runs, I've managed to train for and complete two marathons and an ultra by running three times a week. My approach involved utilising free marathon plans from MarathonPal.com, which detailed how to optimise the limited number of runs. Although it was a challenge to balance family responsibilities and training, I found that prioritising quality runs over quantity was more effective for my body and lifestyle.

Prior to my first ultra, I stumbled upon Bill Pierce and Scott Murr's book *Run Less Run Faster: Become a Faster, Stronger Runner with the Revolutionary 3-Run-a-Week Training Program*. Suddenly, my three-day-per-week training routine made sense. Their marathon plans utilised the same principles I had employed in my previous two marathons. I highly recommend

Run Less, Run Faster to anyone struggling to keep up with traditional training plans and methods. This book enabled me to find a training approach that worked for me without pushing my body beyond its limits, and it helped me prepare for my first ultra race. The key is not to train more but to train smarter. In my experience, running three times a week has numerous benefits, and many runners have demonstrated that excellent results can be achieved by supplementing running with cross-training.

I am always open to trying new approaches in my training. So when I heard about the Maffetone method (MAF), I decided to give it a try. This method involves running at a low heart rate during all your runs, particularly during the base-building phase. Unfortunately, it didn't work as well for me than my approach of running three times a week; I'd say this method is intended for a higher running volume than I was able to achieve. While slowing down has numerous benefits, it ultimately depends on what other activities you incorporate into your training regimen. Instead, I focus on keeping my heart rate in the lower range during my cross-training days. This approach complements my three-day-a-week running schedule and helps me to maintain overall fitness without overdoing it; I can give my body the needed recovery time while still building strength and endurance. This approach allows me to balance my training and avoid burnout, which is crucial for any athlete.

After trying the Maffetone method for a while without much success, I discovered the 80/20 approach, which proved to be a better fit for me. The 80/20 approach suggests that 80%

of your running should be conducted at low intensity, with the remaining 20% reserved for high-intensity sessions.[3] Speed work would class as high intensity. I've also found that doing my cross-training in the low heart rate range aligns more with this approach. Interestingly, Kenyan runners, known for their exceptional running abilities, also train like this: running easy for most of their runs and incorporating intense speed work during the remaining sessions.[4]

I have adapted and customised the 80/20 approach along with my 'running three times a week' method to fit my needs and training goals. I don't always succeed in maintaining a low heart rate for the entire duration when training, but I do my best to try. I believe that each runner should experiment with different methods to find what works best for their body and their goals. The key is to remain open-minded and willing to try new things to continually improve your running performance.

Through my experiences with training for marathons and beyond, I have come to appreciate the importance of making time for exercise, even when my schedule is busy. Consistency and perseverance are vital in achieving great results in running and life. It's important to remember that running should be enjoyable and fun and never become a chore. If you're not enjoying your training, then maintaining consistency and achieving your goals will be difficult. Don't be afraid to try new things and make adjustments along the way, discovering what suits you best (both physically and mentally) through trial and error.

Chapter 22:
Sunday, Runday

The long run is what puts the tiger in the cat.

BILL SQUIRES

I really struggled to get up that morning. I had a busy day ahead, and I knew if I didn't get up straight away, my run wouldn't happen. I stayed in bed for another ten minutes, then I got up, got ready, and took my dog for a walk before running. My watch was acting up again, but I eventually got it to work and headed out. After running 2 miles or so, I looked up and saw a magical rainbow over my running route, moving with me as I ran. If I had stayed in bed, I would have never experienced this – I think the universe had a message for me. I couldn't help but feel grateful for the ability to run and experience moments like this.

Sunday has been my long run day ever since I started running, and there's something really special about it. Occasionally, I run on Saturdays, but it never quite feels the same. I used to have a structured training routine, with set days for running, strength training, yoga, and stretching. But when my son started school, I tried to fit everything around his schedule and stopped running on Sundays, as I felt guilty for leaving my family. Consequently, this made it hard to fit all my runs in during the week and I felt lost without the structure in my training that Sunday runs provided. After a while, I realised that I deserved that special time for myself and decided to bring back Sunday runs to my routine. *Happy mum is a better mum*, I thought.

I wake up early and always try to get up before my son does so I can get myself and my things ready. During the winter, it might be several hours before it gets light, while during the summer, I cherish the quiet mornings when it's already bright out. Usually, I just eat a banana, drink some water as soon as I get out of bed, and then sneak out quietly to avoid waking Jacob, who sometimes ends up in our bed. Soon enough, he'll be too big to want those sleepy cuddles with me, making it even harder to get up and leave him on those early mornings.

My running clothes and shoes were laid out the night before, but it still takes me a while to actually get out the door. I fill my water bladder with water and prepare my hydration vest. I check that I have my gels and salt tablets for longer runs, lip balm for dry lips, tissues for emergencies, and small bags for any trash. I always apply nappy cream to my toes to avoid blisters (especially before long runs), then get dressed and lace up.

Before leaving, I prepare breakfast for my son and get some berries ready for myself for later. When I return, I'll have a simple and easy-to-make breakfast such as porridge, peanut butter, and berries with some plant milk, which works well for my recovery. Variety is important to me, so I like to switch up my breakfast routine with options such as chia seed pudding with goji berries and fresh fruit or yoghurt topped with a combination of berries, seeds, and cinnamon. I love cinnamon!

After kissing my son goodbye, I head out for my warm-up dynamic stretches before starting my run. It's not easy every time. At the beginning of the run, I often struggle to imagine how I'll be able to complete the distance I've set for that day. However, I remind myself that 'it gets easier after 3 miles' and 'I'm doing more than all those people who are still sleeping at home'.

During my runs, I often see incredible sunrises and encounter wildlife such as deer, hares, rabbits, and different birds. Sometimes I even notice the most minor things like a toad on the road; wildlife always brings a smile to my face. I used to run without music, just listening to the sounds of nature. However, these days, I sometimes enjoy listening to music during my runs as it adds variety and gives me something to look forward to.

As my run progresses, I often see familiar faces, such as people who are walking their dogs at the same time. One of them is a friendly farmer who is always walking his dog, Oscar. At first, I was terrified of Oscar as he was always off the lead and would come straight towards me while I ran. I was bitten by a dog when I was nine years old, and since then, I have been cautious around dogs. Although I love dogs, I need to know them before feeling comfortable around them. However, nowadays, every time I see the farmer and Oscar, it gives me a new boost of energy to carry on.

I love seeing people riding their horses during my runs, although I must admit that I feel a bit intimidated by these majestic animals. Nonetheless, it's always a delightful sight, and I often see quite a few of them along my running route. When I run along the riverbank, the sight of swans always fills me with joy. These magnificent birds are indeed a sight to behold, and their grace and elegance never fail to add a touch of beauty to my runs.

I cherish these small but significant moments on my runs, like the sight of rabbits scurrying away at the sound of my footsteps, which never fails to bring a smile to my face. During these runs, I feel blessed. It's incredible how far I can push myself, and it reminds me that I can achieve anything I set my mind to. I love taking in the scenic surroundings and enjoying the peacefulness of early morning runs. Running helps me clear my mind and generates a sense of accomplishment, especially when I cover long distances that many non-runners might find crazy.

The length of my long run depends on where I am in my training: it could be anything from 7 miles to 22 miles. Running longer distances helps me build self-belief and validates perseverance. It may be tempting to give up, but when I set a goal, I give it my all to achieve it. These runs test my mental resilience and teach me to carry on when all I want to do is stop. It's a lesson in stepping out of my comfort zone. No real progress is made if my goals are within my comfort zone. This applies to everyday life as well. When I aim higher, I accomplish great things for myself.

CHAPTER 22: SUNDAY, RUNDAY

Years ago, people who ran marathons seemed like superheroes to me. Running 26.2 miles seemed like an unattainable goal. But now, I am one of them. These long runs have shown me that anything is possible if I put my mind to it. They have helped me untangle my thoughts and provided a sense of triumph that few other activities can match.

Running teaches discipline and commitment and shows us that we can achieve more than we thought. It's also an excellent opportunity to make friends and find inspiration from them. Running cures my body and soul, giving my life a new perspective and encouraging me to make healthier choices. I do most of my dreaming while on my long runs. It's good to dream. As I run, I start to believe that my dreams could actually become a reality.

As I approach the end of my run, I start to think about my post-run routine. I know that when I get home, I'll need to stretch and do some cool-down exercises. I'll also make sure to eat a proper breakfast and hydrate well to aid my recovery.

Finally, I reach the end of my run, and it's a mix of satisfaction and relief. I am proud of myself for sticking to my training plan and pressing on through the challenging moments. I know that the long run is a crucial part of my training and will make me a stronger runner. As I head back home, I am already looking forward to my next Sunday runday.

Chapter 23:
Half Marathons That Changed Me

*Once you make the decision that you will not fail,
the heart and body will follow.*

Kara Goucher

As I write this, a year has passed since my first half marathon. Looking back, it seems both insanely brave and stupid that I ran my first half marathon just five weeks after starting my running journey.

On that day, I didn't plan to run a half marathon. I'd had a big meal earlier, and my knee was hurting (I was struggling with runner's knee at the time). Prior to that day, the longest distance I'd ever run during lockdown was 9 miles. When I set out to run, my initial goal was to hit the 10-mile mark for the first time.

I started my run with a strong pace, and by the time I reached 5k (3.1 miles) and 10k (6.2 miles), I thought I had hit some PBs. My sixth mile was particularly challenging due to strong headwinds, but I was determined to keep going. It wasn't until later that I realised my phone displayed my average pace, not my mile times. Back then, I didn't own a Garmin, and the concept of pace was relatively new to me. Despite the misunderstanding, I was still pleased with my progress, and the feedback I received from the Runkeeper app motivated me to keep pushing on.

When I was just shy of 9 miles, I told myself to aim for 10 miles. The thought then occurred to me that seeing as a half marathon was only 3.1 miles more, I may as well go for it. As I continued to chip away at each mile, I couldn't believe I was running a half marathon. Running a half marathon had been on my bucket list for some time, but I always thought that only 'real runners' were capable of achieving that distance, and I didn't consider myself a real runner yet. Despite the pain in my hips and the fatigue in my legs, I felt a true runner's high.

I continued and felt better the closer I got to the end goal. It was amazing. Just as I finished, I fell and hurt my hands. When I got home, my husband wasn't quite as excited as I was. In the heat of running, I didn't check my phone and didn't see he'd been trying to get in touch with me to make sure I was okay. His reaction made me feel that my achievement wasn't worth much at all. In hindsight, I should have called and told him I would be out longer, but I was afraid using my phone would mess up my tracking. Plus, I wanted to surprise him with my unplanned achievement. I can't really blame him for being so cross, he was just genuinely very worried about me.

I hardly slept that night. There was a mixture of excitement, guilt for making my husband worry, and hunger. I failed to eat after finishing the run, and I didn't eat anything during it either. Running for 2 hours and 34 minutes without any fuel. How naive I was then! My glycogen stores must have been entirely depleted. No gels, no food, just a bit of water, but I did it. It shows that if you eat well before and you're hydrated, you can run longer distances with hardly any fuel (though I wouldn't generally advise it). My pace was slow, but not bad either, considering my fitness at that point. Running a half marathon five weeks after starting running was still a phenomenal success.

The following day, my husband expressed how proud he was of me; I was proud of myself, too! The few races I'd done in Estonia never resulted in a medal (you would receive a goody bag, but no medal). However, this time around, I yearned for tangible recognition of what I'd achieved. I believed that having a medal to hold would make the experience feel more real, showcasing the distance I had run and the effort I'd put in. I had contemplated running a half marathon for years, but never truly believed I could do it. My desire for a medal led me to search for a way my own half marathon could qualify as a virtual race – a concept I wasn't familiar with. While living in Estonia, I participated in a few virtuals, but they did not offer medals. After a brief search, I stumbled upon the website for virtual running, where I could register for a virtual race and receive a medal for the half marathon I had just completed.

So I purchased my first-ever virtual race medal from 'Virtual Runner', which still has pride of place on my medal rack. My husband encouraged me to share my performance and medal on social media, which I did. People congratulated me on the achievement, and I felt really proud of myself. I've since run the half marathon distance many times, but that first time still holds a special place in my heart. It made me believe that I can.

I love a good half marathon distance. I would say it's my favourite. It gives you the feeling that you have run a long enough distance, but at the same time, it's short enough to push for a bit of speed.

One of my favourite half marathons is not my personal best (though it was at the time), but one that changed me. One beautiful Sunday morning, I set out early and after just over a mile, I encountered a mother deer and her two fawns. This close encounter with wildlife was a magical moment that set the tone for a wonderful and enjoyable run. After seeing them, I knew it was going to be a good run. 'It's A Good Day' started playing in my head, and it really was a good day! I set a PB on that joyful, beautiful run. Although that record has since been surpassed, the memory of that particular run still remains with me. Since that first encounter, I have only been lucky enough to spot deer a few more times during my runs. Nonetheless, that initial experience remains a cherished memory.

I managed to achieve my fastest half marathon time under rather grim conditions. The weather was miserable, with incessant rain pouring down, but I remained determined to make the most of the two hours I had before picking up my son from preschool. The run was an emotional rollercoaster, but the prospect of achieving a 2-hour half marathon time kept me going. This run really surprised me. Prior to that day, I had been predominantly doing slow, easy running, and I typically couldn't even complete 6 miles in under an hour.

CHAPTER 23: HALF MARATHONS THAT CHANGED ME • 191

The combination of the music I was listening to and the runner's high helped me battle on. When there were only 3 miles left, I began to feel the weight of exhaustion and the thought of stopping tugging at me. But I refused to give up and strived to get to the end. The emotions I felt during this run were akin to those I experienced during my first half marathon. I couldn't believe it: I was actually going to break my half marathon PB! When I finally reached home, I was drenched to the bone but felt immense pride for having accomplished such a feat.

In 2021, I faced an injury that hindered my ability to run long distances for many months. When I attempted my first half marathon after the injury, I felt a deep sense of gratitude for being able to run once more. I wasn't fixated on achieving a specific time, but instead, I focused on the distance I could cover. Running after the injury felt like a massive achievement, and it reminded me how much I love running.

The half marathon is my favourite distance because it shows that I am on the verge of something bigger; if I can run a half marathon, I know that I can run even further.

Chapter 24:
Runner's High

(noun): An addictive side effect of running, a euphoric state of bliss that may be the reason that runners run.

Unknown

Yesterday's run was a great one, and I was feeling exhilarated. It was interesting how some runs could be better than others. Just two days ago, I had to stop mid-run due to pain, but yesterday I was able to complete the entire 10k without any discomfort. The only difference was that I wore my new trainers. It made me wonder if the wear and tear of winter running had caused my previous shoes to deteriorate faster than expected.

The feeling of elation, or 'runner's high', can be addictive and serves as a reminder that we are capable of achieving our goals. After my latest run, I once again felt that anything was possible, including realising my dream of writing this book. Although this book focuses on my running journey, it also serves as a testament to what I can achieve when I set my mind to it. In the past, I never believed that I could run a marathon, but I did it. Similarly, since I was a teenager I always aspired to write a book, but I needed more confidence in myself to do it. While it may not be everyone's cup of tea, this book is as unique as my running journey has been. I hope that it will inspire and encourage others to pursue their dreams, just as running has encouraged me to pursue mine.

As a teenager, I strived to be exceptional, to stand out from the crowd. But eventually, I realised that being ordinary was a part of who I was, and it wasn't a bad thing. However, that didn't mean that I had to settle for mediocrity. I believe that everyone has the opportunity to achieve their full potential and lead a fulfilling and happy life. To do so, it is crucial to pursue your passions and follow your own dreams rather than those of others.

I believe that endurance sports embody this philosophy. They are the ultimate manifestation of chasing your dreams and proving to yourself and the world that you can achieve them. It's not just about setting fast times but also about pushing yourself to your physical and mental limits. They teach resilience, being comfortable with uncomfortable. One thing is certain: endurance sports change you, and they change you for the better.

I don't experience a massive high from all my runs, but my absolute favourites are my long runs. These runs leave me buzzing with excitement and a sense of triumph. I cherish the feeling of coming home on a Sunday after a long run, being greeted by my son, knowing that I have covered however many miles I set out to do. Each Sunday run is unique in its own way and holds a special place in my heart.

I also enjoy pushing myself to run faster through interval training, which I used to hate. However, I have discovered that a shorter speed session can be just as rewarding as a long run. Today, I attempted a session of 1-minute surges with a 1-minute rest between but struggled to maintain my pace. I found it helpful to choose a landmark ahead and focus on reaching it during my fast intervals, ultimately completing eleven bursts of fast running. I have gained a lot from using the Nike Run Club app's guided sessions. I recommend those to anyone who struggles to do intervals on their own. The guidance from the app helps me remind myself to make sure that I am running with good form during the fast bursts. I also tell myself I look great, and I feel great! Positive self-talk is one of the things that absolutely can make your run.

Running off-road is something that, more often than not, gives me the feeling of runner's high. Being on a challenging surface forces me to be more mindful of my surroundings. Typically, I run slower off-road, which I don't mind as it takes the pressure off. I tend to stick to the same speed across the different sections, which helps me to appreciate my surroundings more and enjoy the run, which is ultimately what it's all about.

Running can be a powerful tool for self-improvement and realising our dreams. The euphoric state runner's high elicits is not just limited to the physical aspect of running but also encompasses the mental and emotional benefits from pushing ourselves to our limits. The feeling of victory and self-confidence that comes with setting and achieving a running goal can profoundly impact our overall well-being.

It is important to note that not all runs will provide the same level of runner's high. Some runs will simply be more challenging. However, it's important to remember that the runner's high is not just about the speed or distance of a run but about the effort put in and the personal progress made. Even a short 2-mile run can provide a sense of pride and boost in mood. Incorporating variety in your running routine can also help to achieve the runner's high. Mixing up the terrain, distance, and pace can keep things exciting and provide new challenges. Speed and interval training can often generate the same euphoria as a long run.

A runner's high is also not guaranteed. Some days, finding the motivation to run may be harder, or the run itself may not gone as planned. It's essential to focus on the progress made rather than the perfection of the run and remember that even a 'bad' run is better than no run. It's also important to listen to your body and not push yourself too hard, as this can lead to injury and burnout.

Overall, the runner's high reminds us of what we are truly capable of; perhaps even something we never thought possible until we tested our physical and mental limits. It's a reminder to focus on our unique progress rather than perfection and to listen to our bodies while challenging ourselves in new ways.

Embracing the runner's high as a bonus of running has a positive impact on our overall well-being and can help us lead a more fulfilling life outside of the running world. Recognising how you can overcome challenges while running fosters further self-belief in our personal and work life, empowering us to tackle obstacles in all walks of life and pursue new dreams with confidence.

Chapter 25:
Tackling the Dreadmill

Time really flies when you're not on a treadmill.

Unknown

At the beginning of February 2021, Paul, my husband, bought a treadmill. He'd had one in the past and loved it, but the only time I'd been on a treadmill was when I went to a running shop to get fitted for my first running shoes. I was sceptical about having one in our small house; I didn't think I would benefit from it and thought it was a waste of money. I had always enjoyed running outdoors, even in bad weather conditions, and didn't want to be confined to the machine.

Despite my reluctance, I decided to give it another try. My ongoing knee injury meant I had recently been experiencing some pain during runs, forcing me to walk for part of them. When I checked the weather the day before my next run and saw strong winds and heavy rain, I knew running outdoors would be challenging. Instead of risking further injury, I opted for the treadmill. I figured this way I'd be able to complete my run and manage my knee pain while still getting another session in.

At first, I felt slow on the treadmill, and every minute seemed to last forever. I found it difficult to pace myself and started too fast, quickly leaving me out of breath, even though my Garmin watch told me I was going at a snail's pace.

After struggling with this pattern for a while, I decided to look into ways to improve my treadmill running experience. I began researching various running apps designed specifically for treadmill workouts and eventually decided to try the Nike Run Club app. Although it was still challenging, it definitely helped me to make progress. However, I still found myself getting bored during my runs and sometimes stopped the workout altogether – something that rarely happened when I ran outside. For me, the main attraction of running has always been getting outside and hitting the pavement. Running indoors just doesn't have the same appeal. Paul, on the other hand, was doing the 'Couch to 5k' programme on the treadmill and thoroughly enjoyed it. He would put his music on and zone out during his runs. I realised that I needed to find a way to enjoy treadmill running too.

I struggled with treadmill runs because I expected to maintain the same pace and effort level as I did outside. It took several treadmill runs for me to accept that running on a treadmill is a different experience; it feels much more complicated, and I find it challenging to run for more than 30 minutes at a time. This was strange for me because, on outdoor runs, a 30-minute jog feels like a warm-up; after 30 minutes on the treadmill, it would feel like I couldn't take another step and needed to get off. I have deep respect for the runners who run on treadmill regularly.

After many not-so-enjoyable treadmill runs through the spring, one morning's run on the treadmill completely changed my perspective and I had my first successful treadmill run! That morning, I laced up my shoes and set a goal to run for an hour on the treadmill. I started the Nike Run Club app's guided 1-hour treadmill run, and instead of using a music playlist that the app recommended, I chose a '80s rock playlist specifically designed for runners. It was a playlist I used on some of my regular runs, as the upbeat music helped me stay motivated and energised. While some of the faster 180 bpm playlists can help to increase my cadence, I enjoy the music less.

It started off feeling easy, but the rolling hills on the treadmill soon kicked in and made things more interesting. During my run, I even pushed the incline button higher than required and finished the guided portion with an intense 12% incline. It was a great feeling to know that I could handle treadmill hills. After completing the guided section, I challenged myself to finish 10k on the treadmill, and I felt great. When I stepped off the treadmill, my face was beetroot red, but the satisfaction was undeniable. This was my first time running 10k on a treadmill, and bonus: it no longer felt like a 'dreadmill'!

Following my successful treadmill run, I began to see the benefits of incorporating treadmill running into my routine, combining it with running outside. Although it wasn't my favourite workout, I started using the treadmill for hill intervals. At first, the transition to and from the treadmill to the road felt a bit awkward, but I soon adjusted to the differences between the two. Now I've come to appreciate the benefits of using a treadmill and attain that same sense of gratification after each run.

Incorporating the treadmill into my training came at a time when I'd been injured for a few months and was unable to log proper distances; I'd begun to lose faith in my ability to run like I used to. With each successful run on the treadmill, I began to feel a glimmer of hope that I could return to my previous running abilities and surpass them. The small victories on the treadmill made me determined to run my second marathon (and perhaps beat my previous time). I even began to think I could attempt an ultra. I was excited to push my limits and see what I was capable of again. It is incredible how a shift in mindset can improve performance.

Chapter 26:
From Virtual Racing to Racing

Those who fly solo have the strongest wings.

Unknown

During my first year of running, I ran solo. My footsteps echoed my thoughts, fears, and challenges. Now, I occasionally run with other people as well and enjoy the company, but running solo is still my first love. Running alone was my sanctuary and for the first six months, I ran without music or earphones and simply enjoyed being alone with nature. The only other sounds I paid attention to were my running app notifications, which alerted me to my average pace and heart rate.

Virtual races became very popular during the pandemic and for new runners like me, it was a great motivation boost and is good practice for future in-person races. For me, a virtual race is as real as an in-person race. The majority of my medals are from virtual races, and I am just as proud of them as I would be if I had received them from in-person races. The distance is still the same. When you run a marathon, whether live or virtual, your body still feels the 26.2 miles. You may still hit the wall. The difference is that there are no crowds to pick you up, no other runners to use as pacers, and nobody to run against the wind with. It's just you and the road and that little voice in your head that lets you know if you can or can't do it.

In fact, even the Boston Marathon has virtual races that are counted towards marathon streaks,[5] and the London Marathon accepts 'good for age entries' (GFA) from the Virtual London Marathon results.[6] A GFA entry means that a marathoner must run a qualifying time within their age bracket either in an officially certified in-person race or in the Virtual London Marathon. Then they can apply for a GFA place in the London Marathon.

Many people argue that running virtual races is challenging since putting in maximum effort is tough without having other runners around you to pace yourself against. However, for me, who wasn't familiar with in-person racing, virtual racing was all I knew. It was my invitation into the running world, and I felt I received the support I needed from other virtual runners.

When I first started running, I only knew a few runners, but through the running club and social media, I have met more and more people who run. My son's teacher is an excellent runner, much faster than me. Occasionally we discuss running and racing at the school gate. Like many club runners, she runs many in-person races. It feels like serious runners are always racing, every weekend and every opportunity they get. I enjoy running, but I'm hesitant about entering races. Part of the reason is that I don't want to sacrifice too much family time on weekends, and part of it is my own hang-up about in-person racing. I feel anxious about the whole thing and I also lack the strong drive to participate, but contradictorily I also fear that not taking part means I'm not a real runner.

I loved the flexibility that virtual racing offered me. I could choose when and where I was doing my runs. Yes, it didn't give me a chance to race against other people in real-time, but I was always racing against myself, not others. I'll never be at the stage with my running where I could win races, and I just want to beat myself.

Virtual racing gives you accountability. You feel that you have paid for your medal and committed to the race, even if it's just you who shows up. It's possible that some people may cheat and submit wrong results, but that shouldn't detract from the positive aspects of the race. In the end, it's just you who you need to beat.

These virtual events allowed me to focus on my own goals and progress; they helped me to become a stronger and more resilient runner. I was able to set goals for myself and participate in races with people from all over the world. It was an excellent way to stay connected with other runners while staying safe at home.

When writing this chapter, I started to think about other people's experiences with running virtual races. For me, running virtual and running solo came naturally. In a way, it was my comfort zone. I admire people who run with friends regularly, but it doesn't always fit in with my circumstances.

During the lockdowns, I asked runners in my Facebook running groups to kindly share their experiences of virtual races; I share a few of them with you below.

Andy shared: 'I took up running in the first lockdown and haven't stopped, although I'm not much better. I had to read and ask lots of questions on forums for tips and work out what running shoes to get after working out that I probably overpronate. Online challenges were also a great introduction for me.'

Sam shared: 'I see a lot of virtual runners who run live events. But I've only just run my first live event. I was a definite virtual running event-only person. I started 4 1/2 years ago because I was fed up with the weight I was carrying. I laced up. My husband asked what I was doing, and I said, "I'm off to do C25K." And that was it. A friend at work told me about virtual running medals, and I became hooked! I'm currently on the injury bench and missing running so much.'

Luke shared: 'As a keen fun runner, I was determined not to let everything stop in the lockdown. Running has the power to boost your mood and well-being. To help me stay active, and motivated and to look after my mental and physical health I have found a great antidote. I have embarked on virtual running, rather than club running, abiding by government social distancing guidelines. The Covid-19 global pandemic has severely impacted charities, but human kindness has been overflowing. The virtual runs enable a percentage of the entry fees to be donated to a designated charity, which has been incredible. It's really satisfying, with this in mind, be kind, don't be put off, have a go, take your first steps and rebuild your healthy habits.'

The evidence from this small group of runners points towards how much virtual running positively impacted them, providing a sense of community, motivation, and a means to stay active during uncertain times. Like them, I found that running and racing solo not only taught me the importance of self-motivation and discipline but also helped me appreciate the support and encouragement of others.

There came a point, however, when more in-person races became available, and I found myself craving the excitement and energy of in-person races. The transition, however, was not an instant shift but a gradual exploration. My first in-person race wasn't technically a race, although it felt very close. It was a running club time trial where we ran without tracking devices. We set off based on our predicted finishing times; the idea was that everyone would arrive at the finish at the same time (in reality it never works, though).

The distance was 7k. I really pushed myself during that run, and I was surprised by how good it felt to compete against other people. No idea about my time, I was pushing myself to run a bit faster. My heart was pounding. I felt a rush of adrenaline surging through my body as I started to overtake other runners, though I wasn't really sure what the etiquette was. As I'd received a lot of encouragement during the run, I tried to offer the same to others. When I crossed the finish line I felt that I was truly a real runner and I wanted to do it again.

Although I still lacked confidence in racing with others, I reminded myself that the more I participated in those events, the easier it would become. I now enjoy the race atmosphere, where you can pace yourself against other people and I get a thrill from overtaking and the adrenaline boost from racing. When you're a rookie to racing, it just takes a bit of time before you start to feel comfortable with it all.

Now, after being a runner for over three years, I feel that virtual racing has served its purpose and I no longer need it. I run for myself, with nothing to prove to anybody. The virtual race medals, sought for my own validation, are now part of my medal rack; tangible proof of what I could achieve. With the pandemic now in the past and in-person races back on, running and racing solo still remains my primary passion – a cherished sanctuary that allows me time for self-reflection and inner peace.

In the beginning, virtual races provided a platform for me to challenge my own limits, to conquer distances I once deemed impossible. When I started running, I couldn't believe I could run 5k. But then I did, and I went on to conquer 8k, 10k, and beyond. Venturing into the unfamiliar territory of longer distances, I needed something to provide that sense of victory you get from crossing a finish line.

Today, having surpassed those milestones, I stand at the intersection of my running journey. The choice to shift away from virtual racing signifies not an end but a transformation – a recognition that I've evolved as a runner. I still run because I can, keeping the inner gremlins at bay and relishing the capabilities my body and spirit possess.

As the sun sets on the virtual racing era of my running chronicles, I step forward, eager to explore new terrains and experiences. Even though I will take part in more in-person races, I will always love running alone. It's my alone time. My serenity. Whether alone on the road or amidst the vibrant energy of in-person races, the essence of why I run remains unchanged – I run because I can.

Chapter 27:
Little Goals Make You Feel Good

Start by doing what's necessary; then do what's possible; and suddenly you are doing the impossible.

SAINT FRANCIS OF ASSISI

Today, I supported my husband running his first 5k. In the past, my running partners were always faster and more experienced than me. However, this time around, I was the more experienced runner, which was a nice change.

Although we were going to run on country roads outside our village, it felt like we were preparing for a race. My husband had recently completed the Couch to 5K programme on a treadmill, and this was his first time running outdoors. While I find running outdoors easier than on a treadmill, my husband felt the opposite. As we got ready for the run, it felt like a proper race day, and despite it not being my run, I felt anxious. This run was incredibly important to my husband, and I wanted to support him in any way I could.

It was just an easy run for me, but my husband pushed himself. And he did it! He ran his first 5k and I couldn't be prouder. It made me feel like I wanted to be part of his next goals. He is now training to run 5k in under 30 minutes. I remember that feeling when I first ran a sub-30-minute 5k, and I really hope I can inspire him to keep running and meet his next goals, and then set new ones.

When I started running, I focused on my own progress rather than comparing myself to others. I would try to run just a few hundred metres further than the last time and gradually pushed myself to run faster. I set small goals for my runs and concentrated on beating my own times rather than comparing myself to others. Running is a personal journey, during which I must face my own triumphs and struggles. It is crucial to prioritise my own objectives and strategies, or I may not achieve them.

As I focused on improving my running time, I discovered how far I could run within 10, 20, 30, or 40 minutes. Sometimes, covering an extra 5 metres in the same time could make a significant difference to my motivation. By running the same route repeatedly, I have become familiar with my pace and distance and can even estimate it without checking my watch.

The last time I participated in a race before I began running regularly in 2020 was back in 2013. It was a women-only race, and although I wasn't in peak physical condition, I managed to run a relatively fast time. I was struggling with a UTI at the time and desperate to reach the finish line so that I could use the toilet. As the race was relatively short there were no Portaloos available on the route, but I persevered nonetheless.

My secret for that race was to run to the toilet as fast as I could; the race conditions might have helped a bit, too.

At the time, I was definitely not very fit. Although I had been going to the gym regularly during the winter, by the time the race came around in May, I had lost most of my fitness. A job I'd started a few months prior was consuming most of my time, leaving me with little time for exercise. I managed to fit in a few occasional runs leading up to the race, but that was all my preparation.

This race time from years ago then became my goal time. What astonishes me is how I was so unfit at the time but managed to run this great time. Even now, after three years of running, I find it difficult to consistently match that race time from the past, though I have managed to reach it a few times. As a result, it is even more rewarding when I can achieve that time or run even faster.

I used to worry too much about comparing myself to others and would get annoyed when occasional runners got better results than me with all my training. But I've learned that we all have our own race to complete and should focus on beating our own times or goals. Running should be enjoyable, and it's important to avoid turning it into a job by constantly pushing to beat PBs. Sometimes it's great to leave the tracking device at home and run at your own pace.

A successful run doesn't necessarily have to be the fastest one. While it's crucial to incorporate some fast running into your training, it's not a great idea to run as fast as you can during every run. There are numerous elements, beyond speed, that you can focus on. You could run while concentrating on different aspects of your running form; keeping your heart rate low; covering a bit more distance than last time; being mindful and simply focusing on feeling good. The options are endless.

During those first few runs in 2020, my goals were simple: get to the next tree, then reach the end of the road, and eventually go beyond 6.6 km (a run from my house). These days, I aim to run 10k or more during most of my runs, but that 10k might be equivalent to your long run. Perhaps you can only fit in a 30-minute run twice a week or you pop on a treadmill once a week when you visit your local gym. Avoid comparing your running mileage to anyone else's. It doesn't matter what your running goals are, what's important is that they are yours and meaningful to you. Your goals are likely different from mine, and they will evolve as you progress as a runner. (For more insights about goal setting head to chapter 33.) Don't let anyone say your mileage is not enough or that you are not a runner if you don't run x miles a week. Remember, if you run, you are a runner!

When you have to step back from running due to injury or illness, remember that you are still a runner; it's just a setback that will make you stronger. It's crucial to adapt your running goals to where you are now. Don't try to run how you used to. Take it day by day and run based on how you feel. Believe in yourself. I believe in you.

Chapter 28:
Running Group

*A comfort zone is a beautiful place,
but nothing ever grows there.*

Unknown

After qualifying as a Run Leader, I had the idea of starting a running group. Although I had joined a running club several months back, I found it difficult to make it to the sessions. With my child starting school and needing my help to adjust to school life, I found it challenging to rush out for a running club session shortly after picking him up from school. Realising that there must be other parents struggling to find time for evening runs, I decided to act on my idea.

Prior to being a stay-at-home mum, I had worked in a challenging and rewarding job that allowed me to use my skills and knowledge to make a difference. Suddenly, I went from being a skilled professional to not working (at least not in a sense of being paid for it; all mums work), which was a significant adjustment for me. While it was great spending time with my son and working on my self-development, I found myself missing any sort of professional challenge in my life.

Fortunately, my supportive husband was there for me throughout this transition. He understands how important it is for me to feel fulfilled professionally and encouraged me to explore different ways to stay engaged and active. During this time, I came up with the idea of creating a local running group for the mums and dads at my son's school. I wanted to use my passion for running to help other parents in the same boat as me to stay active and feel connected while providing a sense of community and support.

Although I'm not exactly a professional athlete, I've learned a lot since I first laced up my running shoes and I felt I had running knowledge that was worth sharing. Starting a running group was intimidating, mind you; I was wondering if I knew enough to lead others. I told myself it's natural to feel scared, but it shouldn't hold me back. I saw it as an opportunity to give back, as running has given me so much, and I wanted to share the joy of it with others.

I decided to start my own group rather than doing it as a part of the running club because I wanted to do it independently and have the flexibility to fit it around my schedule. To be honest, I was also a bit intimidated by the seasoned runners at the running club. Being on my own meant I didn't have to worry as much about impressing others or meeting anyone's expectations; I was solely responsible for my own progress with the group.

It's a liberating feeling to focus on your own goals and to grow as a runner and a leader. At the same time, starting a running group is not without its challenges. There's a lot to consider, from finding a suitable location for your runs to ensuring the safety of your members. You need to have a plan in place and be willing to adapt it as needed. I feel that one of the most important aspects of leading a running group is setting the right tone. You want your members to feel welcome, encouraged, and supported, regardless of their experience level or running goals. It's also important to be open to feedback and listen to the needs of your members.

I knew how I wanted my running group to be, but getting the information out about it took more work than I expected. I asked my child's school for permission to share some flyers, but creating them proved to be a difficult task. I put my heart into it and prepared the flyer, sending it to Paul for feedback. His response: 'It's a good start, but it sounds like an auditor has written it, very factual.' (No surprise really, as I used to be an internal auditor for nearly ten years in my previous life. For those less familiar with the term, an internal auditor is a professional who works within an organisation to evaluate and assess its internal controls, financial processes, and overall operations.) Paul helped me edit the text, making it more engaging and less formal.

The date for the first session was set for ten days after the flyers were distributed. I had already asked some of the parents if they were interested, and some were. The trial session went well, and I found it fun to plan out the weekly sessions. I experimented with different types of sessions; sometimes just going with the flow. It made me feel like a real coach.

When I first attended my running coach course, I was unfamiliar with how running clubs and groups operated, but I had a strong desire to learn. By the end of the course, I had formed a running group and conducted numerous coaching sessions, which significantly boosted my confidence and convinced me that I could deliver effective coaching sessions. I owe much of my success to my little running group.

Starting a running group was a rewarding experience as it created a sense of community, helped others achieve their running goals, fostered personal growth, provided accountability, and allowed for fun and enjoyment. My involvement with the running group motivated me to research and learn more about running, which has helped me improve my own running in numerous ways.

Although I retired our little running group soon after completing my ultra, I find myself reflecting with gratitude on the valuable lessons this experience has imparted. Despite the official disbandment, I still occasionally lace up my running shoes with some former members, fostering the hope that, one day, we will resume it.

Chapter 29:
Rain Rain Go Away Come Back Another Day

―――――――――――

Running any given route in the rain makes you feel 50 percent more hardcore than covering the same route on a sunny day.

Mark Remy

This morning I went for a run in heavy rain. Since I started running, I have become obsessed with checking the weather forecast. I always check the forecast the night before I get my gear ready and again in the morning before heading out. Although the forecast said there was a chance of rain, I thought it would only be a light shower throughout my entire run – not a downpour. Don't get me wrong, I have had many runs where it has rained the whole way through, and I have loved it. In fact, my half marathon PB was in the pouring rain; I got home drenched but happy. I genuinely enjoy running in the rain.

When I first started running, I had quite a bit of figuring out to do. Being short-sighted and wearing glasses for driving, I initially ran without them. The first few times I ran in a downpour without my glasses left me feeling like I was going blind, plus I was wet and uncomfortable. Later, I discovered that running with a cap acts as a little roof, providing enough shelter for my eyes from the rain.

This run was tough to start but got easier as I progressed. At around 10k, I felt pretty good. But then my IT band reminded me that it's still not fully recovered. I tried to carry on, but it soon became apparent that continuing running would only make it worse, and I didn't want to risk a long-term injury.

So I called my husband and started walking. My hands were freezing, and it felt like forever until he arrived and I got in the car. At home, I peeled off my wet layers and took a shower. My fingers hurt so much. When I lived back in Estonia, my fingers were often freezing; I have always had cold hands and feet. But since moving to England, I had forgotten that feeling since it's much warmer here.

I feel like I became less hardcore about running in the rain after my long injury period in 2021. Before then, I would run in bad weather and cold with no issues, but after cutting so many runs short during that spring, I couldn't seem to embrace it as much. Hardly any runs were enjoyable at that point, so why would I go out in the rain? As a runner, you have to be able to run in all types of weather. I felt confident my running in the rain mojo would return soon enough.

Running in the rain can be an empowering experience. It rained a lot during one of our family holidays, so all our activities were planned around the rain. My running wasn't a priority, and I ended up doing most of my runs in either rain or strong winds, or both. As I laced up my shoes while it was pouring outside, my husband asked me, 'You're not going to go out in this?' I did go out. It was hard to start, but then I got used to it. I was dressed appropriately, felt warm, and felt like I was doing a fantastic job of being out in the rain and mud. I am not a big fan of mud, mainly because of the clean-up, but running in the soft mud felt really good.

Four weeks after my second marathon in 2021, I ran my first in-person race since 2013. It was a local 10k race with about seven hundred runners. Along with the running race, there was a military challenge where participants had to carry a weighted pack of 36 lb for men and 24 lb for women; the military entrants set off 15 minutes before the runners. The weather on the day was awful. It had been raining non-stop since the morning, accompanied by strong winds. I arrived at the race where it was still pouring and cold. As we parked up I could see runners everywhere with raincoats or just bin bags on. I was pleased I had stuck to my guns when I packed two bin bags from home. At the time, Paul had said, 'This is ridiculous, no one will wear a bin bag!'

I just said, 'Wait and see, dear.' It's always a great feeling to be right! Most of the participants were freezing as they waited to start running.

The awful weather conditions made the race extremely challenging. It was difficult to maintain a steady pace as I was lashed by the rain and wind, and I had to focus more on my footing than my speed. By the time the hailstones started, I felt truly miserable. I kept thinking, *Did I really pay money to suffer like this?* Several times I thought this wasn't what I'd signed up for and just wanted to go home. I was still determined to finish the race, so I pushed these thoughts to one side.

After struggling with negative thoughts about my ability to finish the race, I put everything I had learned about good running form into practice. Specifically, I honed my arm drive, using it as a focal point to steady my pace and maintain proper form. As I concentrated on this one thing, my negative thoughts dissipated, and I gained confidence with each stride.

It was an out-and-back route, and around the halfway mark, as I was already turning back, I saw some runners I knew coming towards me. Seeing them gave me a bit of encouragement. I managed to get my act together. The hailstones had cleared and the wind wasn't in my face any more. I was able to run a bit faster. Not a lot, but a bit. It still felt incredibly hard, but I told myself I was on my way back now, so it didn't seem quite so bad any more. The distance seemed to go by just a bit faster. When I entered the final 1.5k, I tried to speed up a bit but was worried about running out of energy to finish the race. This is something I struggle with a lot. I know I have more left in me, but I am suddenly conservative and afraid to give everything I've got before the end. When I finally heard that it was just 250 metres left, I let go and sprinted the last stretch.

As I neared the finish line, I saw my husband and son cheering me on. They were both soaked to the bone, but their smiles and shouts of encouragement helped to get me through the last stretch. Crossing the finish line, I was relieved and proud of myself for finishing in such harsh conditions.

After the race, I was surprised to find that I had run a 10k PB. I had wondered whether the race environment would make me faster, but in the end my determination to push through the brutal weather was the biggest factor. I had embraced the rain and hailstones, and it had paid off.

It was a valuable lesson to learn that the most challenging conditions can sometimes bring out the best in us. I may not have enjoyed running in the rain at the time, but it made me feel more hardcore and helped me achieve a personal goal.

From that race on, I was less intimidated by inclement weather. I learned to dress accordingly and was more determined to run through any weather. That was when I reframed my attitude towards running in bad weather or tough conditions: they can be empowering and bring out the best in us as runners.

Despite the pesky setbacks and the temporary loss of my rainy running mojo, I hope that soon I'll be back out there, embracing the rain and reclaiming my love for running in all weather.

Chapter 30:
Canicross

The best running accessory is a four-legged friend.

Unknown

When my dog Stanley passed away, the void left behind was immense. I wasn't emotionally prepared for a new dog, but I missed him deeply. From a selfish standpoint, my son had just started sleeping through the night, and the thought of getting up at night to deal with a puppy's demands was less than appealing. My husband, on the other hand, was eager to fill that void with a new dog. My son missed dear old Stanley deeply and with two votes against one, a schnauzer puppy named Jack entered our lives.

Despite my reservations, I envisioned Jack becoming my running partner. If you know schnauzers, you'll know that behind those gorgeous eyebrows and wise old man look they have a unique personality and stubbornness that can be challenging. As I tried to instil the difference between right and wrong in Jack, it became evident why it's often said that schnauzers become good dogs when they are at least five years old.

I resisted rushing Jack into running and waited the recommended eighteen months before attempting to introduce him to canicross. I also hoped that running would tire him out and he might be better behaved when home. Jack really is a good dog, but when he gets bored (which is often) he gets into trouble. A good schnauzer is a tired schnauzer.

Knowing what a pain in the backside Jack could be I reached out for help. I booked a session with a local lady who offered introduction to canicross sessions. When I started to explore the various gear options, I felt lost and overwhelmed by the multitude of choices available on the internet, not knowing what I would need. I hoped that she could help me figure those things out.

After rescheduling our session a few times the day finally arrived, and Jack and I made our way to it. I didn't know what to expect from it all, so I was nervous and uncertain of how things would turn out for Jack and me. As I turned up in the small car park in my little Aygo with Jack on the backseat to meet her, Jack was confused. Every other time he was put in the car it was either to see a vet or the dog groomer for his coat cut – both options that he hated. And the weather was wet. Very wet. I got out of the car and put on my pink raincoat, carefully packed treats and poo bags in my pockets and hid my phone under my raincoat to keep it dry.

'Hi… Are you Sarah?' I asked the lady who had dogs in her car. By now the rain was getting heavier and it really didn't look great for our session.

'Yes, that's me. You must be Merili. Lovely to meet you,' she answered. 'Do you still want to go ahead with it?' she asked.

'Yes, I am a runner, so a little rain doesn't bother me. The weather forecast promised it will ease up shortly,' I answered … I really hoped the forecast was right.

We decided to carry on in the dreadful weather, and Jack, somewhat bewildered, stood patiently as different harnesses were tried until the perfect fit was found. It's like when we get fitted for new trainers, only his fitting took place in the pouring rain.

Our first run together at our canicross training showed Jack's natural inclination for it. He responded well to basic commands, and by the end of the session I was filled with hope, confident in my ability to tire out my dog, with the expectation that, in return, he would be a well-behaved boy at home. I'd also been told about various canicross gear and accessories. Ever heard of a dicky bag? No, I hadn't either. Basically, it's a fancy insulated bag where you can conceal your dog's poop until you find a suitable bin to dispose of it. I'd never even thought how weird it would be to run around with your dog's deposits dangling from your belt or (even worse) in your pocket, so as soon as I got home I ordered one.

But the next few tries didn't go so well. Jack was triggered by various stimuli during our runs: turning around, passing cars, encountering other dogs. Getting wet or simply becoming excited about running were additional triggers for him. We might have a good run only to endure a horrible one the next time.

A lot of the runs ended with me crying as I called Paul, declaring, 'He's been jumping up on me and nipping again', 'I can't take this any more. I will *not* run with him again'.

I did run with him again. Even with all the struggles, I persevered. Taking breaks, understanding Jack's triggers, and eliminating distractions gradually paid off. Jack, a bit distracted and prone to frequent stops, started grasping the concept. His love for running became evident, and now when I prepare to run without him, he looks at me from under his salt and pepper eyebrows and tries to make me feel guilty for leaving him behind.

In the year since our initial foray into canicross, Jack has truly become a proper running companion. The patience and resilience required for each run became a reflection of the growing bond between us. Our runs turned into a dialogue, with me talking to him and him responding in his unique language.

One memorable run along the riverbank highlighted Jack's preferences – or more accurately, his particular dislike for high grass. As the riverbank stretched out before us, the grass became fairly high in places, providing Jack with a challenge. He trudged through the grass for a mile or so before suddenly stopping and facing me with a look that said 'No, I am not going to run through this.'

I tried to convince him to carry on, but he didn't budge.

'Do you want to go back?' I asked, at which he instantly turned around and eased to his usual trot.

We rarely run on the road. Sometimes time constraints force us to, and if we want to get a run in, that's our only option. One afternoon, we headed out for a quick 5k on the road. The start was slow as always, with Jack sniffing around and stopping a lot. Then he got into it, and we really took off.

When he started to slow down, I gave him a bit of a pep talk. 'You're not a regular dog, Jack. You're an athlete,' I said to him. At first he didn't seem to believe me. But eventually he listened and it really seemed to give him a second wind. We arrived home happy and Jack snuggled up on the sofa for a nap.

I usually run with him once a week, anticipating the surprises and challenges that each new run might bring. With every run I can enjoy his company a bit more. I always talk to him and praise him for his running. When we encounter dogs that once triggered his attacks on me, I remind him, 'Jack, you are here running. You are free, and they are stuck in the garden.' He looks at me and agrees.

Despite the challenges, running with Jack has not only transformed him into a well-behaved canine companion but has also become a source of shared happiness and fulfilment in our lives.

Chapter 31:
Glorious Holiday Running

The obsession with running is really an obsession with the potential for more and more life.

George Sheehan

The first time I attempted a longer distance run was during my first trip to Tenerife. At the time, I wasn't regularly running, but I did have a gym membership and attended fitness classes. For some reason, when I was packing for this holiday in Tenerife I decided to pack my trainers and workout clothes. It was my first time travelling solo, and I had just accepted a new job that was both scary and exciting at the same time. I arrived at my hotel at midnight, eager to explore the area. The following day, I went on a long walk along the beach, on my own, which was a new experience for me – looking back now, I see it took much courage for me to travel solo.

After a delightful morning walk along the beach, I decided to go for an early morning run the next day. This really was an odd thought, because I didn't run at home. On the morning of the run, I had breakfast at the hotel, laced up my trainers and headed out, dressed in capri leggings and a T-shirt. I didn't bring any water with me, but I did bring some money in case I needed to purchase some. As I started running alongside the beach I was surprised by how chilly it was. There weren't many people around, and all the little shops and bars along the seafront were closed. As I continued running, I felt grateful to be running alongside the beautiful beachline. It was one of the most beautiful runs I had ever experienced.

I ran for a full hour before taking a short break to buy a sugary drink which I sipped on as I ran back towards my hotel. By this time, it was around 9 am, and the beach and seafront were starting to come to life as local businesses started to open and more people were out and about. I had about 50 minutes left to run; the temperature started rising and it was becoming quite hot. When I returned to the hotel, I went straight to the breakfast area for some juice before taking a refreshing bath and getting ready for the rest of the day. When I plotted my route on the map I saw I'd covered approximately 10 miles: my longest run ever! (At the time.)

I still don't understand how I was able to run that far without proper training. I hadn't even planned on running that far. It might have been just sheer will and a feeling of possibility that encouraged me to try. I had nothing to prove to anyone. It was just me, without tracking devices, going for an early morning jog.

Inspired by my Tenerife run, when I got home I searched for a half marathon training plan. However, the pressure of the too-fast plan and a feeling I needed to prove something made running tedious. I ran a few times, never quite able to replicate the good feeling I experienced in Tenerife. I eventually stopped running, feeling discouraged by the freezing temperatures and my inability to fully enjoy the activity. Looking back, I realise that I should have allowed myself to run slower and enjoy the process rather than focusing solely on training goals.

Since I started running in April 2020, I've been on several holidays, and all of them have given me great opportunities to run. While I haven't gone abroad for a running holiday yet, I firmly believe that the UK has so much to offer. Yes, the weather can be a bit unpredictable, but the variety of landscapes more than makes up for it. It would be boring if it were always sunny and never rained. As a runner, you really need to learn to run in any kind of weather. It prepares your body for unexpected times: you can't control weather, but you can manage your reactions to it.

My first holiday after picking up running was just a week after completing my first marathon. We decided to stay at a beautiful beach house in Heacham, Norfolk. We arrived at the holiday house in the evening. Jacob had napped in the car on the way there and was extremely excited to be on holiday. It was a bit of a challenge getting everything inside and unpacked, but we managed to get Jacob settled into bed and sort some essentials for the morning. We opened a bottle of prosecco and started to relax a bit. The past week had been all about the marathon – the pre-race excitement and anxiety, the race itself, and the post-race blues. It had been quite an emotional rollercoaster, so it was nice to have some time to unwind.

Despite feeling a bit hungover and tired in the morning, I was eager to run. It turned out to be a glorious run, indeed. After getting dressed and having breakfast, I headed out onto the beach. Everything felt out of the ordinary. I usually never run right after eating, but this time I did, and thankfully I was absolutely fine. My warm-up exercises were the same as they always were, but on the beautiful beach this time. This was also the first time I'd run on sand. It was interesting to figure out which bits of sand were suitable for running on. After less than a mile on the sand, I reached a promenade that was so gorgeous. The sun hadn't risen yet, but it appeared during my run. The stunning views, sunshine, and sea air filled me with gratitude.

I spotted quite a few runners, and, as it was Virtual London Marathon day, I wondered if any of them were running the marathon. I still had that post-marathon euphoria, and I wished I'd had the courage to say to someone, 'You can do it! You can run this marathon!' Of course, I would also mention that I had just run a marathon a week before. I usually don't take photos during my runs, but this time I stopped several times to snap a few. I wasn't aiming for a specific pace, just an easy run, but my pace ended up being faster than expected. I ended up running a glorious 10k that day. When I got back, I was buzzing with excitement and claimed it to be the most beautiful run I had ever completed.

I went on two other runs during that holiday and managed to set a new personal record for my 5k. Before I knew it, I was off the sand and running alongside the promenade. I felt speedy, and it seemed to come out of nowhere. I didn't feel like

I was pushing too hard, but I still managed to complete the 5k at a fast pace, and I'm really proud of myself for that. I think the wind might have helped me that day. This record held for almost ten months; no matter how hard I tried, I couldn't beat it. That run just felt amazing.

I experienced a profound sense of tranquillity during another run on the same time away. I blamed myself for not running my marathon faster, but that day's run reminded me of how much of an impact the wind can have on a run. It doesn't matter how hard you try or how fit you are, headwinds can really slow you down. I wish I'd had more experience with running in the wind before my marathon, as it would have helped me mentally.

My favourite run so far took me to the coast again, this time a few miles from the Lake District, near St Bees. The beach in front of our holiday cottage was a pretty pebble beach, unfortunately spoiled by the amount of rubbish that came in with every tide.

I tried to run on the pebble beach for a bit, but it was too difficult. I was dressed in too many clothes for the weather, and I even managed to have a close encounter with a spiky bush while letting some walkers pass and ripped a hole in my favourite leggings. So my mood wasn't great. After a kilometre or so I considered calling it a day. However, I was still eager for a run, as I wanted to explore the area and have some time to myself. After we had lunch and went for a family walk, I announced to my son and husband that I was going for a run. I really felt like I needed one. I changed my clothes and headed out to the narrow single-track roads. I wasn't thrilled about the new plan, but I hoped that somehow I could make it work.

As I got to the top of the hill, I spotted a sign for the coastal footpath. What a find it was. This run took me over the fields with sheep and lambs. The route had quite a bit of elevation in it, but the beauty of the path made up for it. It wasn't a fast run as you had to open and close gates every once in a while and occasionally let walkers pass. The views, though, were magical. The run ended at St Bees, where it was possible to run further to the top of the hill. It happened to be when the tide was out, revealing beautiful sandy beaches. This run won, becoming an even more marvellous holiday run than my previous favourite. By this point, I was running out of time, so I headed back to the holiday cottage. I was itching to run to the top of the hill and look out for those beautiful sandy beaches again.

Our family had a few great walks on the coastal path, and we all really loved the scenery. I ran the route two more times that week, and on my final attempt, I made it to the top of the hill. It was quite a climb, but I was so pleased I did it. The views from the hill were just as magical as I had envisioned.

Moments like this make me so grateful to be able to run. After struggling with injuries throughout 2021, I appreciate even more when I can run pain-free and have experiences that nourish my soul. Although I cherish my alone time, I would love to share this joy with my closest ones, my son and husband. I hope that one day, we can all run together.

CHAPTER 31: GLORIOUS HOLIDAY RUNNING

Whenever I'm preparing for a holiday, the first thing I pack is my running gear. I've discovered that each holiday destination presents me with a unique 'wow' factor during my runs, and I always look forward to exploring my surroundings through the lens of my running shoes and running while on vacation allows me to immerse myself in the local surrounding and experience the sights and sounds in a more intimate and authentic way. The rhythm of my footfalls sets the pace for my explorations, and with each step, I discover new places and things I might not have seen otherwise. Not only does running during holidays keep me fit and active, but it also helps me appreciate and connect with the beauty of the world around me in a truly special way.

Chapter 32:
Inspiring Movies and Books

Books are the quietest and most constant of friends; they are the most accessible and wisest of counselors, and the most patient of teachers.

Charles W. Eliot

I've always had a deep love for books. I prefer reading physical books over e-books because I adore the smell and feel of paper books. Wherever I live, it's always full of books. When I moved to England, the first items I sent over were my beloved books.

As a child, I was often unwell, but an unexpected positive outcome was that it provided me with the opportunity to read. I liked to explore the different worlds that books had to offer. Although I missed a lot of school, I studied at home and got good grades. The only exception to this was Russian language. I found learning Russian really challenging, and I hated the subject with a passion. To disguise my true intentions, I frequently concealed other books behind my Russian textbooks, hoping to convince my family that I was diligently studying.

But my passion for reading only grew stronger with time. During my childhood, I could often be found in the library, eagerly selecting new books to devour, as well as immersing myself in the ones we had at home. Among my favourites was *Winnetou* by the German writer Karl May. There was something captivating about his vivid descriptions and the characters' almost superhuman qualities that drew me in.

If I couldn't make it to the library I delved into my older sister's mandatory school literature. I developed a deep affection for the books of Erich Maria Remarque (author of *All Quiet on the Western Front*) and the series by Estonian writer A. H. Tammsaare, particularly *Truth and Justice*. The five volumes of *Truth and Justice* explore the protagonist's struggles with the earth, God, society, himself, and ultimately end with resignation. I found solace in the main character's endurance through suffering, which compelled me to read all five volumes.

After my son was born, I just didn't seem to have the time or concentration to read and I just couldn't get into reading any more. It always started well: I chose a book to read but then just couldn't get along with it. It became harder and harder to sit down and concentrate on reading.

Strangely, running gave me back the joy of reading. Running has taught me the value of being present and focusing on the task at hand. As I run, I have learned to tune out distractions and concentrate on the rhythm of my breath and the sound of my feet hitting the pavement. Staying present in the moment helps me overcome physical and mental barriers, gaining a greater sense of clarity and focus both in running and in other areas of my life.

I now always seem to be reading at least one running book at any one time. These books not only teach me about different training techniques and strategies, but they also inspire me to push myself and set new goals. The stories of the people in these books, their struggles and victories, have made me believe that I can accomplish great things as well.

When I first started running, I watched many documentaries in addition to reading books about running. I often think about the people in those stories, their accomplishments, and their struggles. Following their journeys inspires me to pursue my own goals and strive to do my best. I've realised that not everyone runs sub-3-hour marathons, and that's perfectly fine. What's important to me is to be better than I was yesterday. I strive to improve daily, whether by running faster, longer, or with better running form and a lower heart rate.

There are so many people out there doing incredible things, despite the odds. Fiona Oakes, for example, is a vegan runner who runs without a kneecap and has had multiple operations on her knee. She holds several world records for marathon running and is an inspiration to many. For anyone who wants to watch an inspirational running movie or read a book (both are available), Fiona Oakes' *Running For Good* is definitely worth your time.

When you read about running, especially long-distance running, you realise everyone has a story of injury and adversity. But they keep going and accomplish great things. It makes you feel stronger and more resilient. When you feel like giving up, think of all those people who haven't given up. If they can do it, so can you.

As often as I am in awe of the feats of different ultra runners, I am amazed at the undertakings of everyday runners. People on long running streaks, or anyone trying their best to meet their goals, are often even more inspiring. My friend Irene Alisjahbana is one such person. We met in the Facebook group Plant-Based Endurance Athlete just before she completed her eleventh Ironman in four years. She hasn't stopped there and regularly competes, fine-tuning her skills – whether it's in running, cycling, or swimming – to be the best athlete she can be. She is incredibly driven and a great inspiration to me. As mentioned in part I, she virtually ran the last 9 miles with me during my first marathon, which was a great motivator. One day I hope to complete a race with her.

All the books I have read about running have taught me something new and have helped me in one way or another. Ultra runners like Scott Jurek have particularly impressed me. After reading two of his books, *Eat and Run* and *North*, I finally checked out Christopher McDougall's *Born to Run* to dive deeper into Scott's story, who plays a big role in the book. What I love most about Scott is his attitude towards running and other people. He's a phenomenal runner, but he always stays at the finish line to greet other runners. Every runner can learn from both their humble and gracious approach.

Nita Sweeney's book, *Depression Hates a Moving Target*, made me think more deeply about my own struggles with depression. Although my experience with depression has not been as severe as Nita's, running is incredibly helpful for my mental health. I appreciated Nita's honesty in describing her struggles, which included touching on her own experience with incontinence; something many female runners experience but rarely talk about.

Jo Pavey's book, *This Mum Runs*, showed me that even professional runners struggle to find time for training, especially when they have young children. Her story made me feel better about fitting exercise into my own hectic life.

Finding Traction is a movie about Nikki Kimball's ultra running journey, which I found very motivating. Despite struggling with depression, Nikki uses ultra running as her superpower to make it through difficult times. Her determination is truly admirable.

Jonathan Cairns' *Plant-Based Runner* was incredibly helpful when I first switched to a plant-based diet. His book made the transition easier, and his follow-up book, *From Marathon to Ultra*, helped me decide to run my first ultra.

The first running memoir I ever read was Alexandra Heminsley's *Running Like a Girl*. Her straightforward approach to running made it easy for me to identify with her journey. I found it hard to relate to sub-3-hour marathon runners to start with, as I just wanted to complete one, never mind the time! I don't think I will ever be a 3-hour marathon runner, but I *am* a marathon runner. She showed me that it doesn't matter how fast you run; you are a runner.

Some books, like Lisa Jackson's *Your Pace or Mine* and Paul Tonkinson's *26.6 Miles to Happiness*, are simply enjoyable reads that even non-runners would enjoy.

In preparation for my first ultra, I read Rich Roll's *Finding Ultra* and Adharanand Finn's *The Rise of the Ultra Runners*. Both books inspired a helpful mindset for tackling an ultra and helped alleviate some of my anxiety about the race.

While editing this book, I came across Rachel Ann Cullen's three books. What initially began as research on how a well-written running memoir should look soon turned into a genuine interest in learning more about her and her journey. I love her storytelling style and her courage in sharing her challenges to inspire and help others.

Reading about the various struggles and victories of other runners has not only helped me to believe that I can achieve my own goals, but has also helped me to appreciate the hard work and determination of all runners, no matter their level of experience or skill. It's important to remember that we can all learn from each other and support each other in our running journey – wherever it might take you.

You can find a comprehensive list of recommended running books at the end of this book for further reading. Each one has provided me with a valuable piece of my running puzzle or is valued as a great read in its own right.

Chapter 33:
My Top Tips

Nothing is impossible. The word itself says I'm possible!

© Audrey Hepburn

When I first started running, I didn't have a clue how to make it work for me. But through trial and error, I discovered what I needed to do to improve and even enjoy running. Although I made many mistakes along the way, I learned a lot about what works and what doesn't.

Now I better understand what works for me and my body, I'm thrilled to share my experiences with you. However, it's essential to remember that everyone is different, and what worked for me might not work for you. I encourage you to discover the approach that suits you the most. If running isn't your thing, try walking, swimming, cycling, or home workouts. Just be yourself – and remember that you have your own unique journey ahead of you.

The benefits of getting outside and moving your body are numerous, whether it's a leisurely walk or a brisk run. So take a chance and give it a try. Who knows, you might surprise yourself and discover a new passion.

Mind over matter

Goals

You can accomplish anything you want to; you just have to choose to. This may seem like an oversimplified statement, but it holds true. Believing in yourself and your abilities is the first step to success. You will have to work hard, but once you've decided to go after what you want, the necessary training and other steps will begin to fall into place. What may have seemed impossible before will start to feel achievable, and you'll be surprised at what you can accomplish with perseverance and hard work.

When preparing for a race, it can be helpful to set three goals: an optimistic goal, a realistic goal, and a worst-case scenario goal. By having multiple goals, you'll be better prepared for unexpected setbacks.

For my first marathon, I set three time goals:
- Optimistic goal: 4 hours and 30 minutes. Looking back, I realise this was a bit of a stretch.
- Realistic goal: 4 hours and 45 minutes. This was a good goal for me, as I ended up only 2 minutes and 30 seconds slower than this time.
- Worst-case scenario goal: Finish in under 5 hours. This was the time goal that I was determined not to exceed, and it was the one I shared with others as my target time.

Of course, your goals might not be time-related and may differ depending on your experience and personal goals. I have added a handy race pace calculator to the appendices in case you are interested in how fast you would need to run to reach a certain time goal.

For some runners, the goal could be completing the race without stopping, for others only stopping for water breaks; for many runners (especially new runners or those returning from injury), the ultimate goal may be simply to finish the race, which is a great goal to have.

Your why

Your 'why' is the underlying reason or purpose that drives you to complete the challenge. It needs to be personal, emotional, and genuine to motivate you when your body wants to give up. Your initial why may also evolve over time. For instance, if you begin running so you no longer get out of breath in everyday life, this may become irrelevant to you over time once you achieve that goal. Or if you've always dreamed of running a marathon but never believed it was possible, proving to yourself that you can may become your new why. Ultimately, there are no right or wrong answers when it comes to your why – it just needs to be authentic and meaningful to *you*. Identifying your why can give you the extra push to keep going when things get tough. It can also serve as a source of inspiration and motivation, reminding you of your purpose and the sense of fulfilment you will feel when you achieve your goal.

Motivation

Even with the best goals in mind you could lose your motivation. I know I do. I know I want to run, but I feel tired, unfit, and I just don't believe I can do it on some days. One of the things that helps me is wearing a piece of clothing that reminds me of a particularly meaningful performance or good memory. Just putting on one of my old race shirts convinces me I am capable.

What to wear

Clothes

You don't need much specific gear, but there are a few items that you really need. For any item you run in, it's best to avoid cotton as this doesn't wick away sweat, making it more likely you'll suffer from blisters or sore spots. Decathlon is a great place to find affordable running clothes. Women need to invest in a high-quality running bra. Make sure you have a pair of gloves for the winter, even if they're cheap ones; when our hands are cold, we tend to clench them, which tightens our shoulders and affects our running form. Ideally, after a run, change into dry clothes, but if that's not possible, just add a warm layer on top.

It may take some trial and error to discover what works best for you, but eventually, you'll have tested and tried options for running in any weather. Don't rush to buy a raincoat, for example, you'll be surprised how hot you will get wearing one when running. While some find it necessary for colder weather or longer runs, for short, warm, rainy runs, you don't need one. Instead, invest in a good cap; it helps keep water away from your eyes (this is especially important if you wear glasses). Be prepared to get wet and cold during rainy runs, and remember it's important to get dry and warm as soon as you can after your run.

Shoes

For the best fit, I recommend visiting your local running store and getting your shoes professionally fitted. Shoes that are fit for purpose will make a significant difference in your running experience. Once you've been fitted, you can always purchase subsequent pairs online. Many stores carry last year's models, so you may be able to snag a great deal if you're not particular about colour. It's a good idea to periodically get refitted in case your running style or foot shape have evolved over time.

Before visiting the running store, set a realistic budget for yourself. Running shoes are typically the most expensive shoes you'll own (on average £100 a pair), but there's still a broad range of prices available, so if funds are tight, finding a good shoe within a lower price range is still possible.

Orthotics

I have had several pairs of orthotics prescribed, but after initial periods of success, I didn't get along with any of them. Instead, I prefer to use Enertor running insoles for some of my activities as they are soft and flexible and very different from my prescribed ones. In particular, the stiff orthotics that I was prescribed to use did not work well for off-road running. In these situations, I found that my feet needed more flexibility and the ability to adjust to changes in the terrain. So if you plan to do some off-road running, consider using a more flexible pair of orthotics or going without them altogether.

If you use orthotics to correct a specific issue with your feet or gait, it may be best to continue wearing them during all the activities, including running drills, to ensure proper alignment and reduce the risk of injury. However, if your orthotics restrict your movement or limit foot flexibility during specific drills, consider removing them or switching to a more flexible pair of orthotics for those exercises.

Music

When I started running, I avoided music and kept my phone volume up to hear any running app notifications (as I didn't have a running watch to guide me) and to be aware of my surroundings. However, after my first marathon my regular running routes became boring, and I needed a way to spice things up. Initially hesitant to wear earbuds and potentially miss traffic sounds, I tried running with one earbud and loved the extra dimension music added to my runs. Now, I don't always run with music, but I love knowing the option is there.

Before you head out

Getting out of the door

Getting out for a run doesn't always require much time but it does require prioritising your needs and getting creative with your schedule. For parents, utilising support systems is often essential. This may mean running while the kids sleep, but that's okay. The guilt over spending time away from your kids is often overcome by knowing how much happier you are after a run.

To make it easier to get out the door, check the weather forecast and lay out your running clothes and shoes the night before your planned run. This small step can make a big difference and help you feel prepared and motivated. Having everything ready when you have limited time allows you to focus more effectively on your upcoming run.

Planning your sessions

When planning your running sessions, it's helpful to think ahead about the type of workout you want to do, even if you're not training for a specific event. Having a plan provides focus and a sense of satisfaction when you complete what you set out to do.

Safety

Prioritising safety is crucial when running. To ensure your safety, always inform someone of your running route and expected return time, especially if running alone. It's best to run with a partner or group if you can, but if you must run alone, carry a phone with you in case of an emergency. If your watch has the live tracking option, use it. If it doesn't, there are several apps available that can provide the same functionality. You can share your location through WhatsApp or Google Maps, for example.

Wear reflective clothing in low light or night-time conditions to increase your visibility to drivers. Avoid wearing headphones or use bone conduction headphones instead – particularly in unfamiliar or busy areas, so you can remain aware of your surroundings and potential hazards.

ICE tags

When I first started running, I had never heard of ICE tags. The ICE stands for 'In Case of Emergency'. These small tags can be worn on a runner's shoelaces, making them easily accessible and ensuring they are always with the athlete during their activity. These tags are designed to provide vital information in case of an emergency (an accident or medical incident) such as the runner's name, emergency contact information, medical conditions, and allergies. This information can be crucial in helping first responders quickly provide necessary medical care. I strongly advise getting a pair of ICE tags, as they could potentially save your life one day.

Running itself

Avoiding stitch

During my first attempts at running in Estonia (back when I knew next to nothing about running) I struggled to breathe properly and often ended up with uncomfortable stitch. When I found my running mojo in the 2020 lockdown, I knew I needed to address this issue early on in my training. So, this time around, I did my homework. I turned to Google and searched for ways to avoid stitch. To my surprise, the solution was all about breathing. I would practise breathing techniques at home, lying on the floor, focusing on breathing through my nose and into my belly. I even placed a book on my abdomen to visually monitor its rise and fall. It was a helpful drill to prepare for the real situation. Whenever I felt a stitch coming on during a run, I would start breathing deeply, filling my lungs with air, and it helped every time. These days, I rarely experience stitches. Deep breathing not only aids in preventing stitch but also helps me lower my heart rate during lower-intensity runs when I notice it creeping up.

Warm-up and cool-down

As I started studying to become a run leader, I understood the importance of a proper warm-up and cool-down exercises, which until then I wasn't doing enough of. Several injuries later, I realised I needed to change my ways. As a result, I now always encourage other runners to warm up and cool down before and after their runs, and make sure I do the same before my solo runs.

The warm-up is essential to prepare your body for exercise and should follow the RAMP principle. This is a warm-up protocol designed for athletes to prepare their bodies for physical activity. RAMP stands for 'Raise, Activate, Mobilise, Potentiate', which means that the warm-up should gradually raise the heart rate and body temperature, activate the muscles and nervous system, mobilise the joints, and potentiate (or prime) the body for the specific activity to come. By following this protocol, athletes can reduce the risk of injury and improve their performance.

Similarly, the cool-down is necessary to help your muscles return to their pre-exercise state. Start by gradually reducing your running pace to a slow jog or brisk walk. This helps lower your heart rate and allows your body to transition from high-intensity activity to rest. Perform static stretches targeting the major muscle groups used during running, such as the quadriceps, hamstrings, glutes, calves, soleus muscle, and hip flexors. Hold each stretch for 10–15 seconds. Neglecting to stretch after runs can increase the risk of injury, not just while running but also in everyday life.

Running form

One of the reasons I decided to take the running coach course was to improve my own running form. The main issue I faced was frequent injuries due to hypermobility: despite doing all the right things, such as strength training, changing my trainers regularly, taking enough rest days, and cross-training, the niggling injuries persisted. I hoped to find a solution through the coaching course.

I was amazed by the critical role that proper running form plays in enhancing performance and preventing injury; I share such insights and tips below.

The first thing I learned was the importance of a proper arm drive. Adequate arm movement can remarkably increase your speed. Faster arms mean faster feet – your arms, not your legs are your accelerator pedal.[7] Bend your elbows at about 90 degrees and tuck them close to your sides; keep your hands relaxed, your shoulders down, arms low, and focus on pushing your elbows back. The most important thing to remember? Never allow your arms to swing across your body.

You could practise your arm drive with a simple standing arm drive drill. Bend your elbows at a 90-degree angle as you carry out controlled arm swings, simulating the running motion. Focus on smooth, rhythmic movements from hip to shoulder height, engaging the core for stability. This drill aims to enhance arm coordination and muscle memory for an efficient arm drive in running. You could practise it in front of the mirror for instant feedback.

Additionally, running with relaxed shoulders and hands is crucial, as is proper posture: some runners tend to look down while running, but it's essential to keep your head up. Imagine a helium balloon attached to the top of your head, keeping it up. The body should also be erect and straight with no forward lean at the hip. Keep your shoulders relaxed and avoid moving them up and down.

For core and hip positioning, imagine a string attached to your belly button pulling you forward and your pelvis as a bowl of water that shouldn't spill as you run. Imagining these strange scenarios may seem odd, but focusing on even one element at a time can improve your running form.

Foot positioning can be important, and some individuals may experience issues related to overpronation or other foot biomechanics. However, what's more important to note here is how the impact of foot positioning on running varies from person to person. Some of the best runners in the world naturally over or under pronate. If you overpronate or supinate, don't feel discouraged. Appropriate footwear, strength training exercises, and specific running techniques may help address overpronation or supination and contribute to a more efficient and comfortable running experience.

Avoid knocking your knees together: incorporating exercises such as the lateral crab walk, clamshells, side leg raises, and bridges into your routine can help strengthen the muscles supporting hip stability and address this issue.

Increasing cadence is essential for runners, offering benefits like reduced joint impact and improved running efficiency. Optimal cadence varies, but simple adjustments, such as using a metronome or shortening your stride, can enhance performance. Experiment with different techniques and be patient as your body adapts over time.

These were specific tips I picked up during my coaching training. While all of these tips can be helpful, ultimately, it's important to prioritise comfort and freedom during your running. Even if your form isn't perfect, you can still make progress. If you do want to improve your running form, pick one aspect to focus on, perhaps starting with the one you feel needs improving the most.

Running drills

Running drills are exercises that focus on specific aspects of running form and mechanics. These drills can help improve running efficiency and speed, and reduce the risk of injury. Common running drills include high knees, butt kicks, skipping, and bounding, among others.

High knees involve lifting the knees up to hip height while running in place, which can improve knee lift and leg turnover. Butt kicks involve bringing the heels up towards the glutes, which can help improve hamstring flexibility and encourage a midfoot strike.

Skipping involves exaggerated running movements, which can help improve coordination and balance; bounding involves jumping forward while running, which can help improve explosive power. There are various other running drills that you can try, which are designed to enhance different aspects of your running form. YouTube is a great place to find videos demonstrating various running drills; the visual element can help you better understand how to perform these exercises.

I try to incorporate running drills into my training routine as much as possible, usually aiming to do them once a week. However, when time is tight, simply adding some running drills to your warm-up routine can make a big difference. Running drills are a valuable addition to any runner's training regimen, helping to improve form, strength, and overall performance.

Strength training

I have always believed that strength training is an important part of every runner's routine, as it can help improve running performance, reduce the risk of injury, and support overall health and fitness. I have done strength training since the early days of my running venture. By strengthening the muscles, bones, and connective tissues that support running, runners can improve their running efficiency and form, which can help improve running speed and endurance.

Some of the key areas that runners should focus on when it comes to strength training include the core, glutes, hips, and legs. Core exercises such as planks, bridges, and Russian twists can help improve stability and balance. Additionally, glute and hip exercises such as squats, lunges, and hip bridges can help improve power and stability in the lower body. Runners can also incorporate plyometric and explosive movements such as box jumps, single-leg hops, and bounds to improve their running economy and power.

Strength training improves the strength and flexibility of muscles and joints, which can help reduce the impact of running on the body, thereby reducing the risk of injury.

Fuelling

Nutrition

I'm a firm believer in the benefits of a plant-based diet and feel it's the best choice for me. Nevertheless, I acknowledge that individual dietary preferences and needs may vary, and what works best for me may not work for everyone. Regardless of your dietary preferences, it is essential to plan for what you eat. Whether you're running in the evening or first thing in the morning, planning your meals to fuel your body before and after your run is crucial; what you eat can significantly affect your performance and impact your fitness goals.

You will probably need to experiment with different types of food and timing to figure out what works best for your body. While some people may be fine running 30 minutes after a meal, most individuals need more time to digest their food before running. Eating too much or too little before a run can lead to discomfort, nausea, or even fatigue, negatively impacting your running performance.

Some recommended pre-run foods include complex carbohydrates such as oatmeal or sweet potatoes, which can provide a steady energy source throughout your run. It's also essential to stay hydrated and consider adding electrolytes to your water to replenish lost fluids and minerals during and after your run.

After a run, it's key you refuel your body with foods that provide protein, healthy fats, and carbohydrates. Plant-based options such as quinoa, lentils, nuts, and tofu are excellent choices that can aid in muscle recovery and replenish glycogen stores.

One thing I have found particularly tricky is satisfying my sweet tooth without resorting to sugary treats. That's why I'm delighted to share my favourite recipe for vegan chocolate cake, made without any refined sugar. It's simple, delicious, and sure to be a hit with anyone who tries it. So whether you're looking for a post-workout snack or just something to enjoy, try this recipe and see how easy it can be to eat healthily without sacrificing flavour. Trust me: its simplicity makes every bite seem even sweeter.

Merili's little chocolate & banana cake

INGREDIENTS

- Sunflower or coconut oil to grease the tin
- 100 g dried dates (chopped and blended with a little plant milk)
- 175 g self-raising flour
- ½ tsp bicarbonate of soda
- 4 tbsp cocoa powder
- 4–5 very ripe bananas
- 170 ml plant milk (oat milk or soya)

METHOD

Step 1
Heat oven to 160°C/140°C fan/gas mark 3. Grease and line a 2 lb loaf tin with baking parchment.

Step 2
Mash the bananas with a fork in a large bowl. Add all remaining ingredients. Mix well.

Step 3
Gently transfer the mixture into the tin and bake for 1 hour and 20 minutes or until a skewer inserted comes out clean.

Step 4
Cool in the tin on a wire rack. When the cake is completely cool, turn it out onto the rack.

Step 5
Slice and enjoy!

Hydration

As a runner, staying hydrated is essential, especially during hot weather or longer runs. If you're planning to run in hot weather, you need to plan ahead for your drinks. I learned the hard way what happens if you don't hydrate properly during my first 19-mile run when I hit the wall. As a new runner, I had yet to learn how you lose electrolytes when you run, which negatively impacts the body. It was a harsh lesson to learn, but it taught me the importance of proper fuelling and hydration during long-distance runs.

There are numerous options available to keep you hydrated. My preference is to have plain water and salt tablets, but you might prefer a drink with electrolytes already in it. You will also find you need to experiment with different ways to access your chosen hydration. For longer runs, carrying a hydration vest with a water bladder or bottles could be a good option, as it allows you to carry more water without adding extra weight to your hands or waist. Alternatively, a hydration belt with small water bottles could be suitable for shorter runs. Doing loops and having water ready at your house is also convenient for staying hydrated during your runs.

Regardless of your chosen method, it's crucial to drink water regularly throughout your run and not wait until you feel thirsty. Dehydration can lead to fatigue, cramping, and dizziness, which not only affects your running performance but can even be dangerous.

In addition to staying hydrated *during* your runs, it's also essential to hydrate *before* and *after* your runs. Drinking enough water and electrolytes before your run can help you start well-hydrated, while consuming enough water and replenishing your electrolytes after your run can aid in muscle recovery and prevent dehydration.

Alcohol

While I enjoy the occasional drink, I have noticed that consuming alcohol has a negative impact on my running. When I consume alcohol, I am less likely to go for a run the following day, and when I do, I find it harder to put in as much effort as I normally would. Additionally, my heart rate tends to be higher, and I feel more tired during and after my run compared to when I haven't consumed alcohol. Therefore, I believe that less is more in this case, and I prefer to limit alcohol intake in order to maintain running performance.

Rest and recovery

Rest and recovery is vital for athletic performance and overall well-being. When you exercise, your body undergoes stress and needs time to recover. Adequate rest and recovery helps prevent injury, improves muscle strength, and enhances mental and physical resilience.

Getting enough sleep is an essential part of recovery. Most adults need to aim for seven to nine hours of sleep per night especially if you are becoming more active. Rest days (days with no running) are also crucial, especially if you feel exhausted or burnt out. If you can't take an entire day off, try to space out your runs or workouts to allow for more recovery time. Female runners should consider adjusting their training plans to accommodate their menstrual cycle. Some women may experience fatigue or cramps during menstruation, which can affect their training. Planning an easier training load during this time can help prevent burnout and injury.

Engaging in active recovery, such as walking, swimming, or playing sports with your children, can help improve blood flow, reduce muscle soreness, and promote relaxation. Stretching and foam rolling can prevent muscle tightness and soreness. Yoga or Pilates can be excellent options for stretching and strengthening.

Having a sports massage is a great way to alleviate any persistent aches in your muscles, though time constraints and financial considerations mean it's not feasible for everyone to enjoy regularly, so you could consider adding one to your birthday or Christmas wish list – it could make for a wonderful gift. An alternative you can do at home, if you have a bathtub, is to take an Epsom salt bath; it's a wonderful way to relax and relieve muscle tension. I've yet to brave the chill of an ice bath, but it's definitely something I'm curious to test out!

Remember that rest and recovery is just as important as training. Listen to your body and take its messages seriously.

Building up

Increasing distance

When I first started running, I simply went out and increased my distance without much thought or planning. While this approach worked for me at first and helped me discover my love for running, it may only work for some people. This is where Couch to 5k plans come in – they are incredibly popular and effective because they provide a structured approach to running. Most programmes require running three times a week, although some may require more. If you're looking for a sensible way to start running, Couch to 5k is a great option. Alternatively, you can reach out to your local running club for guidance and support. Many clubs offer Couch to 5k courses, and running with others can make a big difference in keeping you motivated and accountable.

Training plans

Countless free training plans are available, and most running books include a section with a set of training plans. While free plans can be great, it's important to find one that suits your needs and make necessary adjustments. Don't become a slave to the plan – if it isn't working, find a way to make it work for you. I spent some time looking for plans based on three runs a week, as that was all the time I had.

Hiring a running coach to create a personalised training plan can be a good option for those who prefer a more customised approach. However, it's essential to ensure that the coach is available to provide guidance and make adjustments as needed during the plan. Real-life events, such as injuries or illnesses, can happen during any training plan, and it's important to be able to adapt accordingly.

In my experience, having a training plan is beneficial, but it's also important to listen to your body and be mindful it is not impacting on your personal life. You can always make adjustments as necessary.

Injuries

Pains and niggles

Injuries can happen to anyone, regardless of their experience level in running. If you feel any pain or discomfort during or after your runs, it's crucial to address it. Ignoring the pain or pushing through it could lead to more severe injuries.

To identify your pain's cause, you should investigate it further. Could it be due to your shoes? Do you need to stretch more? Or are you perhaps overtraining? If you're not sure what's causing your pain, consult with a physical therapist. These professionals can help you diagnose the issue and then develop a treatment plan to address it.

Remember, taking care of your body and dealing with any pain or discomfort during running is crucial for your overall health and long-term running success.

Advice from books

Few runners are immune to pains and niggles, but if you're looking for a comprehensive guide on how to prevent and manage them, I highly recommend Paul Hobrough's *Running Free of Injuries*. This book not only teaches you how to react to any niggles you feel before they become full-blown injuries but also provides a wide range of rehabilitation exercises. For those unable to visit a physio after every niggle, this book will help you get back on the pavement sensibly.

The first-ever running book that I bought was *Science of Running* by Chris Napier. This book covers common injuries and rehabilitation exercises, delves into running form, and introduces you to common running jargon. It includes a list of training plans for different abilities and is an all-round excellent reference book to have. (As for reading for motivation and inspiration, please see recommended reading and also chapter 32 'Inspiring Movies and Books'. There are new books being published daily (like mine!) and I haven't been able to add all the books I have read about running, but these recommendations are a starting point.)

Incontinence

Stress incontinence is a condition that may not be considered an injury, but it can have a similarly crippling effect on those experiencing it. However, unlike injuries, stress incontinence is often not discussed openly, leaving affected runners feeling alone and embarrassed. It tends to affect women more than men, as women's bodies undergo remarkable changes throughout their life, especially after giving birth and the menopause, with stress incontinence commonly viewed as a normal part of life.

As a female runner who had given birth a few years prior to starting running, I have struggled with stress incontinence. It was something I experienced from my very first runs in my garden, making me apprehensive to leave my backyard for a run. During my first year of running, it was a constant worry for me. I tried out different options to manage it and wore a pad for many of my runs. I felt isolated and ashamed of my problem. But after joining women-specific running groups online, I learned that this was a prevalent problem, and I felt less alone and had more courage to seek help.

My situation only started to improve when I sought help from a women's health physio. First, I discovered that wearing a flow cup during my runs reduced my leakage. Then, when I added the Kegel exerciser 'Perifit' to my daily routine, I saw tremendous improvements.

My only regret is not seeking help sooner, but I was too ashamed and believed that stress incontinence was a natural and normal part of being a mum. If you find you also leak when you run (regardless of your gender), I urge you to reach out and seek assistance, while being open to trying various solutions. If you run with a group, remember that you're not alone in your feelings, and there's likely someone else there who shares your concerns or struggles.

Tracking your runs

Kilometres or miles

At the start of this book, I mentioned the utter confusion that arises over whether to refer to your runs in kilometres or miles. As someone who grew up using the metric system, I still prefer to track my runs in kilometres. However, the choice between metric and imperial systems ultimately comes down to personal preference. The most important thing is to use the system that feels most comfortable for you. And if you prefer not to track your runs at all, that's perfectly fine too!

Apps and sport watches

When I started running, I only had a step-counting watch; I had no clue about running apps or fancy sports watches. I ran with that watch for weeks until one day, I decided to measure my distance on Google Maps. It turned out I had been running a lot further than my watch had been telling me! Back in Estonia I used an app called Endomondo, but that had since gone out of business. After some advice from running groups, I tried Runkeeper and loved it, but I struggled with where to store my phone on runs. Then, my husband got me a Garmin Forerunner 35 for my birthday a few months after my first run. It was perfect for me: simple and with excellent battery life, though it lacked the ability to create custom intervals. After two years, I upgraded to the Garmin Forerunner 245, which I love even more than my previous watch.

As for running apps, I've tried several. Nike Run Club app is great for treadmill runs and has some fantastic guided workouts. I mostly use apps to spice up my training and try out new guided runs. Most people have heard of Strava. If it's not on Strava it didn't happen, right? I've never been a big fan of Strava, though. I have an account, but I don't really spend much time on it. I know it might be an unpopular opinion, but I don't believe Strava tells the full story. While I recognise there's a lovely and supportive community out there, especially during periods when running becomes a challenge, I've found myself overly concerned about what others might think of my performance. The pressure to justify my slow runs or returning to running after a hiatus became burdensome. After careful consideration,

I decided to disconnect my Garmin from Strava, and now I feel liberated and in control.

I still share some of my runs on Instagram, but on my terms. I choose which runs to share and when to share them. This shift has granted me a more secure sense of autonomy over my running journey.

Racing

Tapering

If you're going through the taper period before a race, it's essential to prioritise your mental preparation. I didn't feel mentally prepared for how anxious I would feel during the taper period. Engaging in activities like meditation, visualisation, and setting goals for race day can help you stay focused and motivated.

As for diet, I prefer not to make any significant changes before long training runs or a marathon. I stick to my regular routine and consume the same foods I've trained with before. Being plant-based means I already consume plenty of carbohydrates, so I don't need to eat anything special beforehand. I've found that avoiding carb-laden meals the night before and opting for fruits and vegetables works best for me. If I do decide to eat something carb-heavy like pasta or chips, I'll have them for lunch the day before the marathon.

The day before your race is all about packing and checking your things in advance, and prioritising rest and relaxation. You can still be active, but ensure you're not doing anything that may cause additional stress or physical strain. Taking care of your mental and physical state will help you be fully prepared and ready to perform your best on race day.

Packing for the race

Packing for a race can be stressful, but it's important to make sure you have everything you need to perform your best on race day. Some essential items to consider packing include:

1. Running gear – Make sure you have all the equipment you need for the race, including running shoes, socks, shorts/leggings, a shirt or tank top, and a sports bra if necessary. Use Vaseline or nappy cream on any areas that could rub and cause discomfort during the race.
2. Race bib and safety pins – Remember to pack your race bib and safety pins or magnets to attach them to your clothing.
3. Timing device – If you plan to track your time during the race, bring a timing device such as a watch or your phone, and make sure it's fully charged.
4. Nutrition – Bring any nutrition or hydration products you plan on using during the race, such as energy gels, sports drinks, or water.
5. Warm clothing – If the weather is expected to be chilly, bring warm clothing to wear before and after the race, such as a jacket or sweatshirt. Before major races, it's recommended to wear inexpensive clothing that can be easily discarded and you don't mind giving away. These clothes are usually collected by race volunteers and donated to charity. If it's raining on race day, consider

using large bin bags to help keep yourself dry before the race begins.
6. Personal items – Remember any personal items you may need, such as sunscreen, lip balm, or a hat. Just in case, you could bring some painkillers. However, I would only recommend using them if absolutely necessary. It's always handy to take some tissues or toilet paper with you as well. Have some money and your phone with you just in case of an emergency.
7. Recovery items – Consider packing items for post-race recovery, such as compression socks or tights, a change of clothes, and snacks!
8. Spectator items – If you have friends or family coming to watch the race, make sure they have what they need, such as a blanket or folding chairs to sit on.

Overall, thinking ahead and making a packing list is important to ensure you have everything you need for a successful and enjoyable race day experience.

Long runs

Toilet stops

Almost every runner has a humorous toilet story to share – something that has happened to them or their running mates. However, these incidents are a natural part of running, and you shouldn't feel ashamed of them. Mistakes can happen to anyone, whether it's barely making it to the toilet on time, struggling to pull up your pants quickly enough, or accidentally sitting on a fresh pile of dog poop. The last one is a true story shared by a runner when I was volunteering for a 30-mile ultra. While writing this book, I heard some amusing stories proving how almost everyone has had a funny toilet-related incident to share.

If you're planning an off-road running adventure, I have some advice for you: familiarise yourself with the toilet opportunities on the route beforehand. Whether it's a pub, a store, or a friend's house, map out your options ahead of time. If there are no toilets nearby, then bushes might become your new best friend. Just be ready to embrace the natural surroundings and any surprises they may bring!

Sun protection

As runners, it's important to protect our skin from the sun. Trust me, I've made the mistake of thinking I wouldn't be out for long and ended up with a painful sunburn that lasted for days. If you're not careful with your sun protection, you might end up with a fashion faux pas on your hands – or rather, on your legs and arms. Think invisible shorts and running vests, courtesy of your funky tan lines. You might be rocking a cute bikini or swim trunks, but those awkward tan lines will give away your true identity: a hardcore runner who forgot to slather on the SPF. So, before you hit the road or trail, take a minute to apply some sunscreen. It might not seem like a big deal, but it could save you from much pain and embarrassment.

Canicross

When I first considered running with my dog, Jack, I didn't know much about canicross. Initially, I thought I just needed a different lead for it and a belt to go around my waist, and that would be it. However, after a session with local canicross expert (which I described in chapter 30), I gained a wealth of information about canicross. A good starting point is https://dogfit.co.uk/.

First and foremost, you need a well-fitted harness for your four-legged friend. Equally important is the canicross belt *you* wear. Though there are many brands available, I am only familiar with DogFit® gear. What impressed me about their canicross belt was its hip-fitting design, especially crucial when running with a strong dog. A canicross belt that fits around your waist could easily knock you off balance.

During our initial attempts, my dog seemed to have two modes: superfast or stock-still (usually stopping to sniff, and often right in front of me). What surprised me was that although dogs are natural runners, they too need time to progress gradually. Canicross is more of a job for them than simply running around. Additionally, it's essential to consider the surface you run on; a softer surface is better for their paws. While I occasionally run on the road with Jack, I always prefer a softer surface.

As for yourself, ensure you bring a drink for your dog. Many convenient travel dog bottles are available. Personally, I wear my race vest with pockets in the front, carrying my dog's bottle on one side and my own on the other. When it comes to food, it depends on how long you are out for. You can bring snacks for your dog on longer runs, but just like us, eating when running could cause bloating and discomfort. Remember, every dog is different, so it may take time to figure out what works best.

I wholeheartedly encourage you to try canicross if you enjoy running and have an active dog. It's not only fun but also a perfect bonding opportunity for you and your furry friend. If your dog stops frequently, like mine, view it as an opportunity for a low heart rate run. If you struggle to fit both dog walks and runs into your schedule, consider combining them. You don't have to take your dog on every run, but trust me, your four-legged friend will eagerly anticipate those times you do.

Last piece of advice

With the abundance of advice available about running, it's easy to feel overwhelmed. When starting out, it's crucial to begin slowly and gradually increase the intensity and duration of your runs. My approach in the beginning got me the results, but there is a more sensible way. Pay attention to your body's signals and refrain from pushing too hard too soon.

Above all, don't forget to simply enjoy your runs. If you would like to improve your running form, focus on it, one thing at a time. Turn to YouTube and observe how elite runners run. Ask a friend to take a video of your running and try to figure out some easy fixes to focus on during your next runs. As with many things in life, you don't have to have it all figured out at once, but you can make it happen one positive change at a time.

Chapter 34:
Why Run?

Whatever you do, or dream you can do, begin it.
Boldness has genius, power and magic in it.

Johann Wolfgang Von Goethe

I hope that I have successfully conveyed the benefits of running for your fitness and mental health. Follow the tips outlined in this book, and you'll be on your way to a successful and enjoyable running journey. If I still haven't convinced you to lace up, keep reading.

Why run, why bother? I was a different person before lacing up on that sunny April day over four years ago. I didn't believe I could run. I didn't believe I could write a book. I learned a lot about myself through running. This world has given me so much – new friends, confidence, an excuse to spend more time in fresh air, and all those colourful running clothes. It hasn't cured my depressive episodes; running is not a magical cure. However, when my inner gremlins take over and the world seems black and white, I am better equipped to deal with those episodes.

Running gave me a new way to identify myself. At the time when I felt so taken by motherhood, I needed to be someone else than just a mum. While I'm still uncertain who I want to be when I grow up, running has nudged me closer. I'm more at peace with the notion that you don't have to have everything figured out. Goals change; life gets in the way and that's fine. I don't have to aim for the same goals I had three years ago. I am allowed to adjust them to fit with where I am right now.

I have not always been comfortable with meeting new people and entering new situations; interacting with other runners has helped me to be more confident with this. Runners, in general, are a friendly bunch, and it's not often I won't get a hello, nod, or smile back when meeting another runner on my route.

Running has forced me to step out of my comfort zone. I was absolutely petrified when I did the assessments to become a run leader and running coach. I was convinced all those lovely runners who showed up to my sessions knew a lot more than I did. Still, somehow, I conquered those doubts and felt that I belonged.

Somehow, running just helps. I love cycling, both indoor and outdoor, but running still takes the lead. Don't get me wrong, I have experienced really bad runs and limped home crying many times during my injury. But through it all, I never stopped running. I never wanted to.

If you have never run before and you've happened to read my book, please lace up. You won't regret it. Think of all those stupid things I did at the beginning of my running journey, and I survived. There isn't much to lose, only gain.

Maybe you've run in the past and for one reason or another you stopped. I've been there, too. I dipped in and out of running for years before I experienced my own running nirvana. Dig out those old trainers from the bottom of your wardrobe or take that trip to the storage box in your garage; blow off the dust, and lace up. You might not be able to run as you used to. It doesn't matter. You are here today. It's a new start, and all you can do is to show up. Do that and you're already better than yesterday. (And hey, you might want to treat yourself to some new trainers! Especially ones that fit properly …)

If you're considering giving up running because you haven't been able to achieve any new PBs and you feel that you don't even like running any more, try exploring different approaches. Leave your watch at home. Go for a run and count how many red postboxes or dogs you can spot during your run. Just find a different angle. A personal best doesn't need to have anything to do with pace or times. You can work towards a different personal best. Try heart rate training: become frustrated with how much harder it is to run slow, and then find joy in it. Run with a friend and help them achieve their goals. I promise you it will be as satisfying. You can make it work!

And don't let overthinking hold you back – lace up your shoes and go for it! Remember, running is a journey, and every step counts towards your progress. It doesn't matter if you're running for the first time, stepping out after a long break, or trying to rekindle your motivation. It's a new day and a new start. You don't have to run a certain number of days a week or a set mileage. All of this is irrelevant. You do you. Our goals will never be the same, but with dedication and consistency, you can improve your physical and mental health and achieve your running goals. You can do it. Just run.

Running is my refuge when I feel like I'm failing in other aspects of my life. It's my way of feeling better when I'm down. But, most importantly, I run because, well, why wouldn't I?

Epilogue

Experiencing the aftermath of my first ultra was challenging in ways I never could have anticipated. Physically, my recovery was relatively fast. I tried to keep myself moving and focused on active recovery. My running went well for a few months after Dukeries, including a hilly 10-mile race in 28-degree heat.

In September 2022, four months after my ultra debut, I woke up in the middle of the night to drive to Worksop and volunteer at the Robin Hood 100 ultra. I was assigned to the aid station at 84 miles. I hoped that witnessing the runners passing through after enduring a day and night of running would give me a better understanding of what this 100-mile event was truly like. The experience surprised me. I was pleasantly shocked by how fresh people looked as they passed the aid station. In my eyes, everyone who completed the race that day was a superstar. I returned home tired and happy, wanting to run my own 100-miler even more.

Around six months after my ultra I came down with multiple bouts of illness. I tried my best to keep up with my routine, but each time I started to feel better and tried to get back to it, I would get sick again, and the cycle would repeat. Between illnesses, my crippling tiredness just didn't allow me to run like I wanted to. It felt like I was making no progress and I became increasingly demotivated.

I struggled to find the motivation to do anything – not even run or write, which were two activities that typically brought me joy. Depression had set in, a heavy weight on my shoulders that I couldn't shake off.

Months passed, and my exhaustion persisted. I tried different approaches to my training, hoping to find a miracle cure for my fatigue. It seemed like no matter what I did, I couldn't escape the feeling of being trapped in my own body. I felt like I was losing my identity as a runner, and the thought of giving up on my goals began taking root in my mind. On many occasions I felt like I was no longer a runner at all, just an imposter in running trainers.

I visited my GP, who could not find anything physically wrong with me. But I knew something was off. I had lost my passion for running, and even everyday tasks felt like a chore. I knew I wasn't physically injured, but I was struggling. Something was holding me back. My previous marathons and ultra now felt like distant memories, and I struggled to believe that I had once conquered them. I no longer identified as a runner; all I felt was lost and adrift. It was as if I had returned to a place of uncertainty in my life, not knowing where I was headed. Looking back, I believe I had simply become run-down. I was racing to get back to running too soon and not giving my body the rest and recovery it needed.

One evening I started to talk about my non-existent running to my husband and realised that my big dreams were still there. Dukeries wasn't the end of my running journey, the big triumph. It couldn't be. I realised my next goals were still ahead of me. I still wanted to run the Robin Hood 100 in 2024. I had a decision to make. I could carry on sulking and detraining, or I could pick it up and start training for a hundred miler. The idea of pushing my limits and seeing how far I could go was intimidating, but the itch to participate persisted and the tiniest spark of exhilaration ignited within me.

Before I knew it, I was mapping out what the next twelve months of training would look like and I only had one big goal: finish the Robin Hood 100. Making my dreams a reality, however, involved one crucial task. For me, it wasn't simply starting with a training plan. It required a significant shift in my mindset. Once again, I had to silence the inner gremlins and give my running a fresh start. My past personal records and achievements no longer held significance. All I could focus on was being better than I was yesterday.

And so, without further hesitation, I signed up for the race.

Glossary

Back-to-Back Runs: Runs on two consecutive days with minimal rest in between. This approach is often used in endurance training to stimulate fatigue and build mental and physical resilience.

Bone Conduction Headphones: These send sound waves through the skull instead of through the eardrum, meaning you can hear what's happening around you as you run or exercise.

Bounding: A higher intensity running drill designed to improve power and efficiency (a sort of exaggerated running style).

Box Jumps: A plyometric exercise where you jump from the floor onto a raised surface.

Bridge: An exercise where the body is lifted into a bridge position, engaging the core and glute muscles.

Cadence: Is the rhythm or tempo of a runner's stride. It refers to the number of steps taken per minute by a runner.

Carb Loading: A nutrition strategy involving increasing carbohydrate intake before an endurance event to maximise glycogen stores in the muscles.

Clamshell: An exercise involving opening and closing the legs while lying on one's side like a clam, targeting hip muscles. Great to do with a resistance band.

Dynamic Stretches: Active movements where joints and muscles go through a full range of motion.

Electrolytes: Includes minerals like sodium, potassium, and chloride as well as magnesium and calcium; they play a crucial role in maintaining fluid balance and nerve function in the body.

Endurance: The ability to sustain prolonged physical activity, such as running, without fatigue.

Explosive Movement: Quick and powerful movements that require a rapid release of energy.

Fartlek: A Swedish term meaning 'speed play'. Fartlek is a training method that involves alternating between periods of intense effort and periods of easier, relaxed running or walking. It is an unstructured form of training that allows runners to vary their pace and intensity based on how they feel.

Gait: A manner of walking or running.

Glycogen: A form of stored glucose in the muscles and liver, serving as a primary energy source during prolonged exercise.

Half Marathon: A road race covering a distance of 13.1 miles or 21.1 kilometres.

Hip Bridges: Similar to bridges, focusing specifically on engaging and strengthening the muscles around the hips.

Hypermobility: The ability of a joint to move beyond its normal range of motion.

Interval Training: A training method that alternates between periods of high-intensity exercise and periods of rest or lower-intensity activity.

IT Band (Iliotibial Band): A fibrous band of connective tissue that extends along the outside of your leg, from the hip to just below the knee joint. It plays a role in stabilising the knee during movements such as running and walking. Issues with the IT band, such as tightness or inflammation, can lead to discomfort or pain, particularly on the outside of the knee.

Kegel: A pelvic floor exercise involving the contraction and relaxation of the pelvic muscles used to control urinary flow.

Lactate Threshold: The point at which the body produces lactic acid faster than it can clear it away.

Lactic Acid: A chemical your body produces when your cells break down carbohydrates for energy. It can feel like a burning sensation in the muscles that are working hardest.

Lateral Crab Walk: A lateral movement exercise where one moves sideways in a squat position. Best done with a resistance band.

Lunge: A lower-body exercise where one leg is positioned forward with the knee bent while the other leg is extended back. Great to help tone and strengthen quads, hamstrings, glutes and calves.

Marathon: A long-distance race with an official distance of 26.2 miles or 42.2 kilometres.

Metatarsalgia: A condition in which the ball of the foot becomes painful and inflamed, often associated with running or high-impact activities.

Negative Split: Running the second half of a race faster than the first half, resulting in a negative split time.

Pace: The speed at which a runner is moving, measured in minutes per mile or kilometres per hour.

Pain Cave: The physical and mental dark place that athletes enter during intense physical exertion, like ultra running.

PB: Short for personal best, the best time or performance achieved by an individual in a specific race or workout. Also referred to as PR (personal record).

Plank: An isometric core exercise where the body is held in a straight line from head to heels, typically supporting the body on the forearms and toes for the maximum possible time.

Plant-Based Diet: A diet based on foods derived from plants, such as fruits, vegetables, grains, and legumes, with little or no animal products.

Plyometric Movement: Exercises that involve rapid contraction and extension of muscles, such as jumping and bounding.

Pronation: The natural side-to-side movement of the foot during walking or running.

Neutral pronation: Feet naturally roll inwards up to 15%.

Overpronation: Happens when your gait (the way you walk or run) eventually causes the arches of your feet to flatten more than they would normally, causing your ankles to roll inwards more than 15%.

Underpronation (Supination): Outward rolling motion of the foot during walking, where the foot fails to roll inwards enough to distribute the impact evenly.

Reps (Repetitions): referring to the number of times a specific exercise is performed in a workout.

Runner's Knee (Patellofemoral Pain Syndrome / PFPS): A common overuse injury causing pain around or beneath the kneecap.

Russian Twist: An exercise involving twisting the torso while seated or lying down, often done with a weight.

Salt Tablets: Oral supplements containing salt, commonly used to replace electrolytes lost through sweating during intense exercise.

Shin Splints (Medial Tibial Stress Syndrome / MTSS): A common condition characterised by pain along the inner edge of the shinbone (tibia).

Side Leg Raises: An exercise involving lifting one leg sideways while lying on one's side, targeting hip muscles.

Single Leg Hops or Jumps: A plyometric exercise that helps in developing power, simultaneously improving balance and stability. Single-leg jumps can help you increase your vertical jump by increasing the speed at which you can move your body up, then down again.

Single Leg Squats: Single leg squats help strengthen leg muscles and improve stability. When doing one, ensure your knee stays aligned with your middle toe, lowering yourself as far as possible without letting the knee drift inward towards the big toe side.

Squat: A strength exercise in which the athlete lowers their hips from a standing position (as if sitting down) and then stands back up.

Static Stretches: These require moving a muscle as far as possible (without feeling pain) to improve muscle flexibility.

Stress Incontinence: Involuntary leakage of urine during activities that put pressure on the bladder, such as coughing or exercising.

Strides: Short, fast runs, often around 100 metres, performed to improve running form, increase leg turnover, and enhance speed.

SWOT Analysis: A strategic planning tool used to identify and evaluate the Strengths, Weaknesses, Opportunities and Threats involved in a project.

Tapering: The reduction of exercise volume and intensity leading up to a race or important event. Tapering typically occurs in the weeks leading up to a race, with a gradual decrease in mileage and intensity.

Tempo Run: Also known as a threshold run, a tempo run is a workout performed at a comfortably hard pace, just below the lactate threshold. It's a pace that's about 25–30 seconds per mile slower than your 5k race pace. You should be able to maintain this pace for at least 20 minutes and up to 1 hour.

Ultra Marathon: Any footrace longer than the traditional marathon distance. The shortest common ultra marathon is 50k or 31 miles.

VO2 Max: A measure of how much oxygen the body can consume during maximal effort. Most running watches calculate a runner's estimated VO2 max.

Appendix 1:
Recommended Reading

Books about how to run

1. Scott Douglas. *The Little Red Book of Running*. Skyhorse Publishing 2011
2. Lexie Williamson. *Yoga for Runners: Prevent Injury, Build Strength, Enhance Performance*. Bloomsbury 2023 (second edition)
3. Matt Fitzgerald. *80/20 Running: Run Stronger and Race Faster by Training Slower*. Penguin 2015
4. Paul Hobrough. *Running Free of Injuries: From Pain to Personal Best*. Bloomsbury 2016
5. Chris Napier. *Science of Running: Analyse your Technique, Prevent Injury, Revolutionize your Training*. DK 2020
6. Carrie Jackson Cheadle and Cindy Kuzma. *Rebound: Train Your Mind to Bounce Back Stronger from Sports Injuries*. Bloomsbury 2019
7. Julian Goater and Don Melvin. *The Art of Running Faster*. Human Kinetics Publishers 2012

Books about why we run

8. Christopher McDougall. *Born to Run: The Hidden Tribe, the Ultra-runners, and the Greatest Race the World has Never Seen*. Profile Books Ltd 2010

9. Jonathan Cairns, Caleb Cairns and Fiona Cairns. *From Marathon to Ultra: How Someone Ordinary Gets to do Something Extraordinary*. JC Runs 2021

10. Scott Jurek. *Eat and Run: My Unlikely Journey to Ultramarathon Greatness*. Bloomsbury 2013

11. Vassos Alexander. *Don't Stop Me Now: 26.2 Tales of a Runner's Obsession*. Bloomsbury 2016

12. Nita Sweeney. *Depression Hates a Moving Target: How Running with My Dog Brought Me Back From the Brink*. Mango Media 2019

13. Alexandra Heminsley. *Running Like a Girl*. Cornerstone 2013

14. Lisa Jackson. *Your Pace or Mine?: What Running Taught Me About Life, Laughter and Coming Last*. Octopus Publishing Group 2016

15. Anna McNuff. *The Pants of Perspective*. Rocket 88 2017

16. Jo Pavey. *This Mum Runs*. Vintage 2016

17. Jonathan Cairns. *The Plant-Based Runner: A Personal Guide to Running, Healthy Eating, and Discovering a New You*. Independently published 2019

18. Paul Tonkinson. *26.2 Miles to Happiness: A Comedian's Tale of Running, Red Wine and Redemption*. Bloomsbury 2021

19. Scott Jurek. *North: Finding My Way While Running the Appalachian Trail*. Cornerstone 2019

20. Adharanand Finn. T*he Rise of the Ultra Runners: A Journey to the Edge of Human Endurance*. Guardian Faber Publishing 2020 (second edition)

21. Rich Roll. *Finding Ultra, Revised and Updated Edition: Rejecting Middle Age, Becoming One of the World's Fittest Men, and Discovering Myself*. Random House 2013

22. Rachel Ann Cullen. *Running For My Life: How I built a better me one step at a time.* Blink Publishing 2018
23. Rachel Ann Cullen. *Running for Our Lives: Stories of everyday runners overcoming extraordinary adversity.* Vertebrate Publishing 2022
24. Bella Mackie. *Jog On: How Running Saved My Life.* HarperCollins 2018
25. David Servan-Schreiber. *The Instinct to Heal: Curing Depression, Anxiety and Stress Without Drugs and Without Talk Therapy.* Rodale Press 2004

Books about plant-based eating

26. Matt Frazier, Matt Ruscigno. *No Meat Athlete, Revised and Expanded: A Plant-Based Nutrition and Training Guide for Every Fitness Level—Beginner to Beyond.* Quarto 2018
27. Katy Beskow. *15-Minute Vegan: Fast, Modern Vegan Cooking.* Quadrille Publishing Ltd 2017
28. Gaz Oakley. *Plants Only Kitchen: Over 70 Delicious, Super-simple, Powerful & Protein-packed Recipes for Busy People.* Quadrille Publishing Ltd 2020
29. TJ Waterfall. *The Plant-Based Power Plan: Increase Strength, Boost Energy, Perform at Your Best.* Penguin 2021

Appendix 2:
Miles vs Km

Miles	KM	Miles	KM
1	1.61	16	25.75
2	3.22	17	27.36
3	4.83	18	28.97
4	6.44	19	30.58
5	8.05	20	32.19
6	9.66	21	33.8
7	11.27	22	35.41
8	12.87	23	37.01
9	14.48	24	38.62
10 🏅	16.09	25	40.23
11	17.7	26	41.84
12	19.31	26.2 🏅	42.2
13	20.92	31 🏅	50
13.1 🏅	21.1	40 🏅	64.4
14	22.53	50 🏅	80.47
15	24.14	100 🏅	161

Appendix 3:
Km vs Miles

KM	Miles	KM	Miles
1	0.62	24	14.91
2	1.24	25	15.53
3	1.86	26	16.16
4	2.49	27	16.78
5 🏅	3.11	28	17.4
6	3.73	29	18.02
7	4.35	30	18.64
8	4.97	31	19.26
9	5.59	32	19.88
10 🏅	6.21	33	20.51
11	6.84	34	21.13
12	7.46	35	21.75
13	8.08	36	22.37
14	8.7	37	22.99
15	9.32	38	23.61
16 🏅	9.94	39	24.23
17	10.56	40	24.85
18	11.18	41	25.48
19	11.81	42	26.1
20	12.43	42.2 🏅	26.2
21	13.05	50 🏅	31
21.1 🏅	13.1	64.4 🏅	40
22	13.67	80.47 🏅	50
23	14.29	161 🏅	100

Appendix 4:
Race Pace

1 Mile	1 K	5K/3.1 Miles	10K/ 6.2 Miles	10 Miles	½ Marathon	Marathon	31 Miles/ 50K
05:00	03:06	15:32:00	31:04:00	50:00:00	01:05:33	02:11:06	02:35:21
05:30	03:25	17:05:00	34:11:00	55:00:00	01:12:06	02:24:12	02:50:53
06:00	03:44	18:38:00	37:17:00	01:00:00	01:18:39	02:37:19	03:06:25
06:30	04:02	20:12:00	40:23:00	01:05:00	01:25:13	02:50:25	03:21:57
07:00	04:21	21:45:00	43:30:00	01:10:00	01:31:46	03:03:32	03:37:29
07:30	04:40	23:18:00	46:36:00	01:15:00	01:38:19	03:16:38	03:53:01
08:00	04:58	24:51:00	49:43:00	01:20:00	01:44:53	03:29:45	04:08:33
08:30	05:17	26:24:00	52:49:00	01:25:00	01:51:26	03:42:52	04:24:05
09:00	05:36	27:58:00	55:55:00	01:30:00	01:57:59	03:55:58	04:39:37
09:30	05:54	29:31:00	59:02:00	01:35:00	02:04:32	04:09:05	04:55:09
10:00	06:13	31:04:00	01:02:08	01:40:00	02:11:06	04:22:11	05:10:41
10:30	06:31	32:37:00	01:05:15	01:45:00	02:17:39	04:35:18	05:26:13
11:00	06:50	34:11:00	01:08:21	01:50:00	02:24:12	04:48:24	05:41:45
11:30	07:09	35:44:00	01:11:27	01:55:00	02:30:45	05:01:31	05:57:17
12:00	07:27	37:17:00	01:14:34	02:00:00	02:37:00	05:14:38	06:12:49
12:30	07:46	38:50:00	01:17:40	02:05:00	02:43:52	05:27:44	06:28:21
13:00	08:05	40:23:00	01:20:47	02:10:00	02:50:25	05:40:51	06:43:53
13:30	08:23	41:57:00	01:23:53	02:15:00	02:56:59	05:53:57	06:59:26
14:00	08:42	43:30:00	01:27:00	02:20:00	03:03:32	06:07:04	07:14:58
14:30	09:01	45:03:00	01:30:06	02:25:00	03:10:05	06:20:10	07:30:30
15:00	09:19	46:36:00	01:33:12	02:30:00	03:16:38	06:33:17	07:46:02
15:30	09:38	48:09:00	01:36:19	02:35:00	03:23:12	06:46:23	08:01:34
16:00	09:57	49:43:00	01:39:25	02:40:00	03:29:45	06:59:30	08:17:06
16:30	10:15	51:16:00	01:42:32	02:45:00	03:36:00	07:12:37	08:32:38
17:00	10:34	52:49:00	01:45:38	02:50:00	03:42:52	07:25:43	08:48:10
17:30	10:52	54:22:00	01:48:44	02:55:00	03:49:25	07:38:50	09:03:42
18:00	11:11	55:55:00	01:51:51	03:00:00	03:55:58	07:51:56	09:19:14

References

1. Chris Napier. *Science of Running*. Dorling Kindersley 2020
2. Nita Sweeney. *Depression Hates a Moving Target*. Mango Publishing 2019
3. Matt Fitzgerald. *80/20 Running*. Penguin Group 2014
4. Adharanand Finn, 'Kenyan Lessons', https://www.tracksmith.com/gb/journal/article/kenyan-lessons
5. https://www.baa.org/virtual-125th-boston-marathon-fact-sheet
6. https://www.tcslondonmarathon.com/enter/how-to-enter/good-for-age-entry
7. Julian Goater, Don Melvin. *The Art of Running Faster*. Human Kinetics 2012

Acknowledgements

This book would never have existed if I had never laced up and headed out for that first run in April 2020. Despite how challenging the Covid-19 pandemic and subsequent lockdowns were, I am grateful for the push it gave me to get off my backside and take that crucial first step.

Enormous thanks to my editor, Siân Smith from Sian Smith Editorial. I had been working on my book for a few years and I was in a state of doubt when I stumbled upon Siân's Instagram account by chance. She sounded like someone I needed, even though I wasn't looking for an editor at the time. When I saw her post about a last-minute editing slot, I sent her a message. We didn't waste time and jumped onto a discovery call a few days later. I booked her there and then. Siân believed in me and my writing and with her help and support I was able to bring the project to completion.

She was the one who really looked at my manuscript with a fresh pair of eyes and gave me suggestions that made my book the best it could be. I am truly grateful for all the hours she has put into working on my book.

Special thanks to fellow running coach Steve Portess from TeamBR for his invaluable advice on running form, drills, and strength training sections of the book. Your expertise is deeply appreciated. Having completed a running coach course together, I can attest that there are few coaches who consistently learn, challenge themselves, and develop as you do.

A heartfelt thank you extends to my first readers, Irene, Paul, Rachel, Gina, and Sarah, whose feedback was invaluable. It took me a lot of courage to share my work with you. I vividly recall the anxious wait as my first reader Irene delved into my manuscript. Her feedback was instrumental in ironing out initial inconsistencies, often overlooked by the author. Gina and Sarah, I am grateful for you taking the time to read parts of my book and providing me with feedback and encouragement. Rachel, thank you for being my friend and always happy to support me as I figured out the different elements of writing the book.

I spent many hours at playgrounds and soft plays with my son, allowing my husband the chance to read my book. All feedback was highly valued and spurred me to work harder to improve my writing.

Gratitude goes to Rob Payne and everyone at the Caistor Running Club who assisted me in obtaining my certification as a run leader and running coach. As a newcomer to the club, I was warmly welcomed and received help with my assignments.

Thank you to the club members who were present when I completed my first ultra – you made the finish truly special. And you certainly know how to make running fun!

Thank you, Laura, Angela, Gemma, and everyone who joined me for the running group sessions and helped me to become a better coach and runner. You forced me to step out of my comfort zone and played a crucial part of my learning.

Appreciation goes out to everyone I've run with and connected with through running. I've gained valuable lessons from each of you. Special thanks to my non-runner friends who have listened to me talk about running and been there for me when needed.

The most heartfelt gratitude goes to my dear husband, Paul, for supporting me through the highs and lows of writing this book. You believe in me even when I don't believe in myself, and I couldn't have done it without you.

Lastly, Jacob, thank you. I run to be the best mum I can be for you and to show you that you can achieve anything you dream of. I love you with all my heart.

About the Author

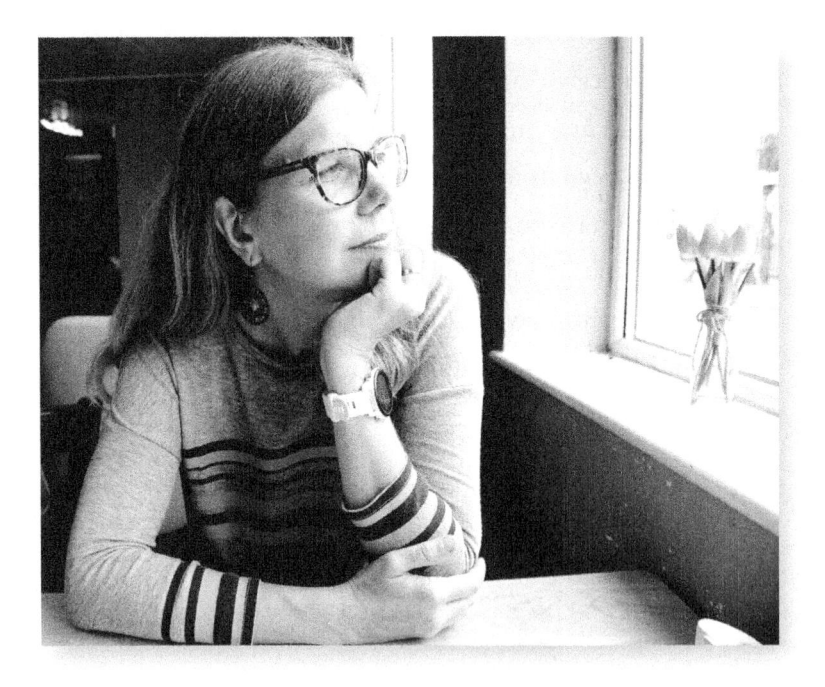

Merili Freear began running in April 2020 during the first Covid-19 lockdown in England. Since then, she has run many thousands of miles, including two marathons and an ultra marathon. Through her experiences, Merili has learned that it's possible to achieve things that may seem impossible at first glance.

ABOUT THE AUTHOR

Merili mostly runs alone and cherishes the positive impact it has on her mental health. Running solo has taught her that anything is possible and that our bodies are capable of much more than we think. Moreover, it has taught her that our minds are powerful tools, especially in endurance sports. It's all about being comfortable with being uncomfortable.

Though she treasures her solo runs, Merili actively engages with the running community, recognising the power of shared experiences. Within a remarkably short time, she achieved England Athletics LiRF (Leadership in Running Fitness) and CiRF (Coach in Running Fitness) qualifications.

Just Run: Discovering my love for running and how the impossible becomes possible is her first book and was written to inspire others to lace up their shoes and head out for that first run. She believes that running can enrich your life in many ways.

Originating from Estonia, she now lives in rural Lincolnshire, England, with her super supportive husband, son, and crazy schnauzer, Jack.

Connect with Merili and share your running experiences by dropping her a line at meriliruns@gmail.com. Follow her running adventures on Instagram (@meriliruns).

Printed in Great Britain
by Amazon